The YIPPEE KI-YAY Principle

Or: The 'Old Black Cloud' And How To Outrun It!

By

Leonard McClane

Cover Design by Mark Flaherty
(www.meandalan.cc)

For my wife, who taught me how to live.

And my beautiful boys, who gave me a reason to.

"... It's difficult to accept the difference between who you are in your head and who you are in the world."

- Abe Applebaum

The Kid Detective

"Helping one person might not change the whole world, but it could change the world for one person."

- Anon

Contents

Part Three

Preface:
The DIE HARD Principle

The book you're reading now was a different book in its initial creation. For one, it had a totally different title more obviously aligned to its concept. You see, the first draft of this book was called 'The Die Hard Principle' – a self-help book / memoir that intricately used the movie Die Hard as a working analogy for our mental health issues, the impactors and our tools to overcome them. There were script excerpts partnered to the points and examples I was trying to make around stress, depression and the like. There were screenshots from the film used as illustrative points too.

And when the book was completed and I'd handed a manuscript of it that I was happy with off to trusted and constructive readers within my friendship group, I put in a licensing application to Disney (who now own 20th Century Studios, were once more famously known as 20th Century Fox and who produced and distributed Die Hard and its sequels under that studio title). I put it in with *such* confidence that it would be approved that I went ahead and roped in the wonderful Mark Flaherty from the Me & Alan graphic design company to design what turned out to be a fantastic book cover for it (and who'd been responsible for the much complimented cover art for my three fiction books – Lehman's Terms, Lehman's Run and Lehman's Infamy; still on sale now!).

After all, what company is going to reject a self-help book for people suffering with mental health issues?

Especially one which has designs on eventually having a portion of its royalties signed over to specific mental health charities and support services?

They licence Die Hard Christmas ornaments and calendars. They let Die Hard characters get printed onto all sorts of t-shirts and jumpers. There's Die Hard colouring books and games and...

Disney refused to let me use the title for the book. Or any direct dialogue quotations from the script. Or any screenshots from the film or cover art font that could be associated with it. And, while they were at it, they rejected my use of imagery and speech from the movies The Verdict, My Cousin Vinny and any other movie I'd used for illustrative purposes in the book that now fell under the 20th Century Studios umbrella, because they own them too.

Their reason was not given outside of the fact that they don't have to provide one. And their decision was final. Mickey Mouse shut the door in my face whilst Goofy held me down and Donald Duck set fire to my manuscript. One of my good friends believes I was rejected because I spoke ill of the Die Hard sequels. I think it's because back in 2002 I littered in Disneyland Paris and now I'm on some sort of blacklist.

You think I'm kidding? My mate Richard once tried to take a baby buggy into Disneyland in Florida that was wider than 79cm and the incident that ensued as a result was such that now he bursts into tears every time his wife tries to log into Disney+ to watch Grey's Anatomy. (Seriously, look up the buggy rule. It's a real thing. They don't fuck around, man.)

Anyway, come on now. This is only the Preface. Let's stop getting distracted:

If there's one thing you'll come to take away from this book it's that I don't give up.

At least not easily.

Sometimes to my own detriment.

Okay... *often* to my own detriment.

My own wife once threatened to divorce me if I didn't stop meeting personal barriers and rejections in our lives with a rally cry of "We don't quit – We recalibrate!" after she got sick of shouting back that my attempts to make that rhyme were driving her insane.

My drive to get this book out there in the hope that my story, my strategies and my beliefs around mental health could help just one person was so strong that I didn't quit. I recalibrated and the book that *was* became the book that *is*.

God, how pretentious did that sound?

The screenshots went into the bin. So did the direct quotes. And obviously the title too. Mark Flaherty stepped up and recalibrated the cover art. But the story, strategies, beliefs and core purpose of the book remain identical. There'll be the odd moment here and there where I may pay reference to something that was once overtly placed in the original attempt of the book. Overall, though, it's ostensibly the same book but with less pictures – and a different title. Some have even said it's a better one. You can decide.

I just hope you enjoy it and get something from it regardless.

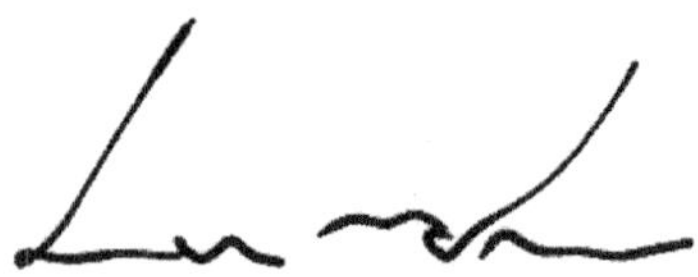

Leonard McClane

Part One

Introduction:

The YIPPEE KI-YAY Principle

Let's get the awkward stuff out the way immediately, yeah?

If you're looking for "definitive answers", "easy fixes" and the like then I'm not your guy and this is not your book. I'm just a bloke who's dealt with depression and mental health issues for so long now that I've not just nicknamed them all under one banner ("The Ol' Black Cloud") I've developed different strategies, tactics and techniques over many, many years that have finally worked for me and I would like to share them with you.

I'm not medically qualified. I have no background in psychology, psychotherapy, counselling or any other 'head doctoring' – other than as a frequent "customer", so to speak. And it's from *that* position that I'm putting this book forward to you. I've been around the block with a myriad of depressive episodes and mental health issues, and I've found some things that worked, some things that didn't, and I've found that throughout the entire 'journey' the biggest asset whether when accessing counselling, treatment or medication has been total transparency and absolute honesty – with yourself, with your GP and with any support services you're accessing.

You can take up some of the stuff I throw your way and use it yourself. You can look at these things, scoff and say "Pfft. I'm not doing that." You can do some. You can do all. It really is up to you as to what fits, what feels comfortable, etc. You can even just read it for the film recommendations whilst inwardly thinking "I'm not taking mental health advice from someone who uses words like 'myriad'!" if you like?

The way I look at it is this: When it comes to taking recommendations on holidays, you always favour the comments from the person who's been where you're thinking of going don't you? When it comes to the realities of war, you're likely to take the word of the solider who's just back from the war zone over the kid who has only ever experienced it on Call of Duty 8 or whatever, right? Well, I've done many all-inclusive trips to the island of Depression, and I've done many tours of duty over in Stress, Anxiety and Post Traumatic Stress Disorder. And I'm happy to take your questions?

The aim of this book is a simple one – I just want one person to feel less alone and for the monumental feelings that their mental health may be causing to feel less singular through talking about my own. I want even just one person to read this book and think "Oh, I thought I was alone in feeling like that!" or "Well, I've never given that a go when it comes to my depression / stress / anxiety / etc!" and "I've never looked at that in that way before, maybe I'll try that!"

I should set my stall out first and foremost by explaining that everything I discuss with you will come from a position of being someone who believes that depression and any other mental health illness is something that is not actually *cured*. Controversial, I know. It isn't the mental equivalent of Athlete's Foot where there's a cream or a spray that sorts it out (though if my own Athlete's Foot is anything to go by, that's never actually cured either!). I believe issues around trauma, stress, anxiety, self-esteem, addiction, PTSD, paranoia, loneliness, and depression aren't "fixed" in the sense that they go away and they're *gone*. I believe that they're there in us and remain in us, a part of what makes us who we are in a lot of ways and that they're simply 'managed' rather than 'cured'.

One of the ways I believe that such things are 'managed' is by cultivating a sense of control around them.

So that it is *us* who influence and regulate these mental health issues, and we are at our worst mentally and/or emotionally or at our most poorly when it is *the issues* that are in control of us.

The clearest way I defined my own depression was in regarding it as a 'black cloud' that is always up there, floating around above me somewhere. And that to not get wet (i.e. depressed) when it unloads on me is to functionally stay one step ahead of it.

If you read the words "wet" and "unloads" and did like a little Beavis & Butthead chuckle to yourself, I can assure you that you're going to enjoy this book and we're going to get along. If that was a bit too base and juvenile for your tastes, worry not one jot because I also use more words like "myriad". I think I use "plethora" at least three times. And "ostensibly". There's something for everyone, I promise.

How I stay ahead of the proverbial cloud is what I want to share with you and for you to see if it helps you do the same or similar with what is affecting you. I'm not going to be using worksheets with old-fashioned clipart in it that makes you feel a bit infantilised, don't worry. I'm going to be doing it through discussing films with you and suggesting you look at those films and see if you feel the same way about them – or more importantly *they* make *you* feel something.

I'm going to get you to look at your best and worst thoughts and see how you feel about them when you've 'went to town on them' a bit. That's about it. This isn't the book that's going to have chapters with inspirational quotes as headers. You know, like *"Winners do what losers don't want to!"* and *"Wasting time is robbing oneself!"* Or *"To read without reflecting is like eating without digesting!"* Nor are we going to summarise what we've learnt in this section or that section by signing off with stuff like *"Remember, understanding yourself is the best path towards understanding others."* Or *"Don't forget; the best preparation for tomorrow is doing your best today."*

This isn't that. I promise.

I am probably going to use the word "journey" a lot though.

I think it is only fair to warn you in advance about that. I apologise.

This book is going to be chatty bullshit around a subject as vast, complex and often upsetting as mental health. Who knows exactly what this book is? Self-help textbook? Memoir? Both? *Neither*? I guess as long as it doesn't end up being described as a "manifesto" on the evening news whilst they show a really unflattering photo of me on screen then we're okay, right? We're going to be using films as metaphors and maybe as teaching tools in some instances.

Yeah, I'm totally serious.

Come back. Honest, it could be fun. Who knows?

Let me give you an example of what I mean:

It's like the film, Die Hard. You know Die Hard, right? If you've not seen Die Hard I think you may well have bigger problems at play than this book can help you with. But I'll humour you: It's a 1988 John McTiernan action film now regarded as a masterpiece of its genre, the father of an entire subgenre of 'Die Hard on a...' knock-off action thrillers (see: The Rock, Cliffhanger, Sudden Death, Passenger 57, Air Force One, Con Air and Under Siege) and an adoptee of the "Classic Christmas Film" label (Die Hard *is* a Christmas film – there's no room here for alternative points of view on this!).

Bruce Willis plays a New York City policeman called John McClane who heads out to Los Angeles somewhat reluctantly to visit his estranged wife (Bonnie Bedelia) and two children. He catches up with her initially amidst the annual Christmas party at her place of work, only for terrorists to interrupt the festivities and take everyone inside the LA skyscraper hostage. After acting as an intermediary to the ineffective police and specialist services taking position outside fails, McClane reluctantly realises that the only person who's going to be able to save his wife, protect the hostages and keep him alive is... himself!

And get this: Within this metaphorical act of whimsy that you're going with me on, **you're** McClane! The terrorists are your mental or emotional ill-health. The police are your psychiatrists, psychologists, counsellors, etc. The SWAT team is your medication(s) and the like. You've went to them. You've leant into them to "save the day". But they're not working or they're not effective on their own, they're not going to come into play in enough time, something like that. It's on *you*, McClane. You've got to step up and take charge here. Let the "police" strategise outside, or whatever. You must go get the shit done.

The metaphor stretches – Maybe you're not *entirely* alone. Maybe your medication helps just a little bit but doesn't necessarily help enough? Maybe your counselling worked for a time but you're feeling you've plateaued with it, or it's come to an end too soon and you are neither entitled to more for free nor able to afford more privately? In which case, you're in Die Hard With A Vengeance territory. That's the third film in the Die Hard franchise, in case you didn't know. There are five films though most pretend there's only four. True blue Die Hard obsessives like to pretend there's only three, but that's a whole other thing for another time. Stop distracting me please.

In this 1995 action sequel, McClane is in the process of divorcing, he's suspended from the police force and he's an alcoholic. But when a terrorist (Jeremy Irons) attacks New York City and draws him into a deadly game of 'Simon Says', McClane has to team up with his colleagues and a streetwise cynical civilian (Samuel L. Jackson) to affect a heroic counter-attack and save the city. It's the same Die Hard formula but this time round McClane has other people helping him to get the shit done. Regardless though, shit ain't getting done until McClane puts down the booze and gets his arse into gear.

Getting serious for a second, what I want to do with this book is help you recognise that there may well be help out there but if it's not working for you or it's not going to get offered to you with any modicum of recency, it's about time to lean in on that feeling that you've tried everything else in terms of external help and start tapping into looking internally and making really *small* adjustments to your life that can often help in ways other things haven't. This book is about perhaps looking at how you're feeling a little differently, finding little signs and cues out there that you're not alone in how you feel or what you're struggling with. (I'll be using films as my 'cues' in case you haven't noticed?)

Whichever Die Hard film you go to as a frame of reference – and I'm reminding you there really is only *three* Die Hard films for the purposes of our mental health journey – it was not that the help wasn't ostensibly out there for McClane, it was that he recognised against the odds he was faced with the help wasn't going to be sufficient enough or provide the needed solution quick enough and that it was on himself to step up and take control.

Hell, I buy this Die Hard principle so mightily I forged my penname after the main guy in the movie(s). C'mon, what does that tell you?

And what does "stepping up" look like, exactly?

If we're to believe my theory that mental health is an illness that stays with us and is never truly cured definitively, and that successfully 'treating it' lies in our control of it within our lives, then to apply my 'black cloud' analogy once more there isn't anyone out there moving our legs for us to stay ahead of it. That's on *us*. Help may point us in the right direction to put the best amount of distance between ourselves and 'the black cloud' but it is on us to get there.

That's what this book is about – the methods that helped me 'Die Hard' my way forward when I reached a point in the road where I felt no help was coming and the help that was wasn't particularly effective to / for me.

It's a 'private space' in book form for you to learn a little *from* me and apply some of the smaller things that worked for me and hopefully may work for you too. It's about passing the proverbial ladder back down, in a lot of ways. You might think you've done the whole therapy thing, or you've tried setting personal goals, but maybe you've not tried them *this way*? It's a twist on the traditional and with some unique 'takes' from the perspective of someone who's lived, survived, and endured through it and is talking to you from a first-hand standpoint not a medical one.

Listen, I never thought I'd eat a Spaghetti Bolognese with baked beans in it until I met my wife. I remember looking at the plate the first time and thinking to myself "No fucking way!" But I gave it a tentative try and... now I won't eat Spaghetti Bolognese unless it's made by her because Spaghetti Bolognese with baked beans in it is bloody *delicious*!

Mental Health, Movies and Me - Part 1

I was born to two parents who did not want me or to put it more accurately initially wanted me for reasons people should not generally have children but then were very quickly disappointed by me. And told me so. Regularly. And from a young age too. When you start out in life being told you're a disappointment, it can cause some... *problems*, shall we say? We'll get into the whole 'roots' thing a little later but for now, let me assure you it causes problems!

What sort of problems? The 'quick rundown version' would encompass an absence of complete self-worth for the first three and a half decades of my life, deep depressions, suicide attempts, self-harm, toxic relationships, mental health collapses (i.e. 'nervous breakdowns') and destructive choices. All whilst my parents stood off to the side making statements like "You're always blaming us for your problems!" whilst I was profoundly confused and routinely hurt by the fact that all attempts made to win what I perceived to be their respect or their validation only led to depression, suicidal inclinations, self-harm, breakdowns and so on and so forth.

My father was a man who had some minor celebrity in his teenage years as a professional footballer scooped out of school and put on track to being trained for big league clubs.

He didn't get formal qualifications from school as he was on his apprenticeship with Such-and-Such FC from fourteen. He was a paid professional footballer soon after and lived the life from 15 of typical sportsmen of that era; drinking, smoking, carousing with women and rolling out to play every Saturday.

Before he had even turned twenty years of age he was injured in training after a prestige signing with the biggest club in the region and his football career was over in the blink of an eye – spat out onto 'civvie' street with no money saved, a chip on his shoulder and no discernible skill set or qualifications that could net him a paying job. Through my grandfather's assistance as a 'union representative' my father got in on some low-paying, menial, manual labour job but that 'chip' on his shoulder (as in major resentment and anger at his status in life) constantly got the better of him and he bounced from job to job through all of my childhood; either a victim of redundancy time and again or victim of his own temper for lashing out at someone at work that saw him swiftly paid what he was owed and shown the door.

My mother was born one of two sisters within a strict upbringing by my maternal grandfather, who was a lovely man that did not suffer fools one bit. She was a highly competitive woman with a deep inferiority complex that saw her constantly judge herself and her successes against other people. It was a complex she would project upon the whole family as I grew up – you didn't do anything for the enjoyment, you did it to attain positioning as the 'best'. She wanted the best things in life at a material level and considered the grand achievement in said life to be marrying, getting a job, working your way up in that job, owning your own home and looking to your left and right at all times to make sure that your job, your home, your car and so forth was *superior* to the people you were positioned between.

My mother wanted children because her parents instilled upon her that this was what happened once you were married and settled, and on top of that her friends within her social circle were having children and becoming the centre of attention and my mother would not have liked that. My father did not want children. He liked the freedom of finishing work, hitting the social club after his shift, coming home to his tea on the table and having his weekends for more drinking and taking my mum out. He did not want to have a child get in the way of that.

My mother wore him down and as a result my sister was born. My mother was happy. My dad was happy she was happy and as far as my father informed my paternal grandparents, that was that. Within two or so years though my mum became 'rattled' that all her friends were now having second children and she thought she should too. My maternal grandparents coaxed my dad round by insinuating it could be a boy and then he would have someone he could train in the football opportunities my own dad missed out on. My paternal grandparents allegedly stood off to the side, reserving comment but later said to be somewhat concerned because they did not see my mother and father as 'natural' parents with one child and worried what the pressure of two would bring. (My grandmother in fact told me that they never thought about bringing a second child into their own family because of how difficult my father had been to raise, and she thought the same way about my sister; a very needy and demanding child who would destroy a day if she wasn't the centre of attention in it at all times.)

My mum told family that she 'had' to have a second child because she loved her first so much that she was endlessly troubled by anxiety around losing her and then having *no children* so she thought she should have another one "just in case". This was apparently her final word on the matter as to how I ended up being conceived against my father's better judgment. Weird, right? Well, hold up. One, yeah, I think that's a very weird rationale to make for having a child if you're not a member of the Royal family. But two, apparently the iconic filmmaker Brian DePalma grew up parented by a mother who told him he was a "mistake", and his middle brother was in fact the "just in case" baby. He was allegedly superfluous to requirements. So... yeah, there's a lot of *weird* out there huh?

My parents tired of me very quickly.

I was around eight years of age when I recall they first called me "weird". I liked to draw and make my own comics, and I could do so for hours. They hated this and hated it even more when I would attempt to share with them what I had created.

They saw no value in it whatsoever.

My father was such a cliché that he would on occasion walk into my room and pull the pencils or felt pens from my hands, put a football in their place and tell me to get outside. He would frequently burst into my room and swipe the Lego I was playing with off my table or bed and shout for me to stop being "weird" and "get outside with [my] friends"!

Any form of creativity of any kind was just unacceptable to my parents. The older I got the more brazen they became in diminishing its value; telling me again and again that people like me didn't make money "writing and drawing stories", which was a weird thing to be saying to a ten or eleven year old. My mother would routinely take the approach of explaining that these interests of mine would get me nowhere because it was "too hard" to get a job and support a family doing "silly things like that". My father refused to attend any school play I featured in because he said it was "embarrassing" and would tell family within my earshot that he thought I was "growing up gay" and that I lived in "Cloud Cuckoo Land".

My dad was highly regarded locally as a youth football coach, and he became quite well known for cultivating kids into big talents. There are several professional footballers that are either in the game now or have moved into managing premiere league football teams at this very moment that started out at ten or eleven years of age on my dad's team, under his tutelage. I was not good enough to make the cut for any of his teams. I wasn't that interested in doing so anyway. But every year, like clockwork, he would have me try out anyway then cut me from his final line-up whilst a parent of one kid would inevitably make some variation on the remark "God, how bad do you have to be not to get a sympathy slot on your own dad's team?"

Eventually my parents started to lose interest in me and any sort of push towards the sporting arena. On training nights, they would go rent me whatever they deemed suitable from the local video shop and leave me home alone with that film and all the doors locked. On game days they would send me to my paternal grandparents for Sunday lunch where I'd spend my time curled up on the sheepskin rug in front of the electric fire. This move backfired enormously on my parents and my relationship with them:

The more they distanced themselves from me, the more my grandmother would shore up that distance with love and my grandfather would do the same with the sort of teachings normally reserved between a father and a son. The more they leant on hastily acquired video tapes to serve as 'babysitter' the more I found an escapism from my life at home and an even stronger interest in storytelling and creative arts.

I grew up with film not just as entertainment but as a comfort blanket and a teaching tool. I grew up seeing my grandmother and grandfather as closer to being my parents than my own parents. And my mother and father *hated* that with a passion. They were happy in their relationship with my sister and how she was growing up within the mould they wanted for her. They were very unhappy that I was not doing the same and saw my grandparent's cultivation of my interests and personality as a barrier and a handicap.

My parents frequently dealt with their unhappiness towards me with acts of violence. The violence was couched in screamed statements of my wrongdoing, and I grew up into adulthood believing that the things they did to me were things that parents did to all children when they'd "crossed the line". I was in my early thirties and in the fledgling stage of a relationship with my now wife before I would learn that this was not the case.

I thought the way my parents 'went on' was just a variation of what all parents did. I was actually in counselling - describing a time when my dad caught me reading a biography of Freddie Mercury and held me down and beat me about the face and head with the book whilst shouting that I wasn't going to grow up to be a "faggot" – when the person I was talking to said "You describe that in such a matter-of-fact way that it worries me you think it is in some way proportionate or acceptable?"

The bodily scar I still have from my mother driving a high heel shoe through my skin because I couldn't swallow soluble aspirin? The first time I had my nose broken and it being by my father? The displaced rib cage from a kick to the stomach from him because I tried (and failed) to clean our tropical fish tank? It's genuinely amazing how you can sell yourself on the idea that you're deserved of such things for so long. But then it's amazing how much you can get away with against someone when you raise them with no self-esteem.

Let's side-track a second and delve into self-esteem in more detail. It's such an intrinsic part of my mental health journey it kind of behoves me to lay some solid foundations around it, don't you think?

Self-esteem – or self-confidence / self-worth to some people – is how we perceive ourselves. It's the value we give ourselves as a human being and it's based on our own beliefs regarding how we see us as the person we are. Therefore, if our beliefs or opinions have been hijacked or damaged in some way by a poor episode of mental health and the like then you can imagine how A becomes affected easily by B.

Self-esteem is incredibly important and a damaged form of it or more importantly an absence of it can be very, very affecting upon us.

We need it to feel that we matter and that we are good enough, to be able to move past mistakes we have made whilst proportionately holding ourselves to account fairly, and most significantly we need it to like and value ourselves as people and recognise the strengths we have to offer.

We often must be kind to ourselves for a variety of reasons and an absence or low volume of self-esteem can prevent us from being able to do this because it is very easy to believe you are undeserved of such kindness if you don't have that feeling of self-worth.

There are several factors involved in causing low self-esteem or a complete absence of it. This can range from being bullied, having problems at work, physical problems such as a weight gain or a dilapidating injury, relationship issues, money woes and unrealistic expectations being bestowed upon you by outside influences. I grew up with my family being an issue in this regard. Society has it far worse now because of social media.

Self-esteem issues in and of themselves are not mental health problems but they are causation factors around mental health. A lot of medical professionals believe low self-esteem can be signage towards a mental health ailment. Some see mental health difficulties as being a cause of low self-esteem, especially when length of time is factored in. There is only so long a person can hate themselves or feel so utterly hopeless and worthless. I should know. Think of the relationship between mental health and self-esteem as a circular river that routinely flows round into itself.

The first time I thought about killing myself I had just turned 14 years of age. It was coming up to Christmas and I had been taken to the hairdressers by my mother for my 'Christmas Cut'. I was still not allowed to choose how I had my hair cut / styled, even at that age. The haircut was a disaster and I looked ridiculous with this flat-top 'Ivan Drago' style that I did not suit at all. We were due to go to a Christmas party for my dad's football club that night and I returned home to much mockery from my sister and my father about my new haircut. In anger at one of my sister's remarks I kicked her ghetto-blaster (hey, remember ghetto-blasters?) and it broke.

I was slapped so hard that I banged my head off the door frame and got a lump above my eye. My mum did not want to explain away the lump, so I got banned from going to the party that night and left alone in the house under the pretence of a "punishment".

The door got shut and locked, and I sat alone in my room a week or so out from Christmas looking at my reflection in the mirror and feeling nothing but hatred for myself.

I didn't like how I looked, and I didn't like who I was because the way I figured it I must be bad if my own family didn't like me. I looked out the window at the wrong moment and I saw two lads from my school walking through the snow outside with their arms wrapped round the waist of two girls from my class – and I was so jealous.

I wanted that but I knew, or felt I knew at all of fourteen, that I would never get it; my mother was always telling me my skin was too bad, my father was always telling me my posture was too awful and my sister was always telling me my interests were "too weird".

Who would want to walk in the snow in the early evening of a Saturday night with me? I was too ugly and too strange. What was the point in me living because everyone else was having so much fun and *none of this* was fun to me?

Those were some ***huge*** thoughts and feelings to be having at fourteen years of age, don't you think? Looking back at this moment in time, I wish I could reach through and put my aged hand on my younger version's slouched shoulder and tell him it is going to be okay. I well up writing this because it seems like only yesterday that I had this feeling and yet I'm thirty-plus years separated from it at the time of recounting it to you now.

No hand came through the vessels of time from the future though, and I'd probably have died of shock (or subsequently ran out and bought stock in Apple) if it had. Instead, I reached a point of deciding that I wanted to die.

And I knew exactly how I was going to do it too – dressing gown cord around the neck, other end tied to the banister, step off the banister ledging... jobs' a good 'un!

But just before I got started, I noticed that The Last Starfighter was just about to begin on telly. And I *loved* that film (I still do!).

For a kid growing up with no self-esteem, the idea that there was a world where you could get swept up and away from your meagre existence and told that you were an important factor in saving the galaxy – well that was just some *great* escapism right there.

Catching sight of the TV Times magazine my dad kept on the arm of the chair (no matter what my mother projected, we were not a rich enough family for us to be able to afford the bumper [then-classier] Radio Times festive edition), I saw that straight after The Last Starfighter another channel was showing Mike Hodges' [much maligned then but beloved now] Flash Gordon. And wait! *Later*, there was a Billy Crystal action film I hadn't heard of called Running Scared and after that was Escape From New York, which I had once watched at a sleepover and loved.

I looked at the clock on the wall and realised that by the time my parents had arrived at the venue, got set up, hosted the party, cleaned up and travelled home again in the early hours I could watch all four of these films almost back to back. Undisturbed. And to top it off, as an act of 'revenge' against my family for hurting me and leaving me behind I was going to eat their Christmas 'supplies'. That's right; I scooped up every selection box, my dad's expensive honey-roasted peanuts jar, my mum's 'best' mint chocolates... I spread them out on the carpet in front of me and I ate, ate and ate *some more*. Between films I would go upstairs, vomit then come downstairs and delve back into the food.

I prepared for double punishment upon their return.

When I heard the car on the drive in the early hours of the morning and my family come through the door, I lay in bed pretending to be asleep, but I clenched my fists regardless knowing that a beating was coming.

I heard my mum screech from the bottom of the stairs about what I had done. I heard my dad on the landing outside my bedroom door. My mum demanded he got me up and I heard my dad somewhat drunkenly sigh then mutter "Just leave it. Just leave it. I'll replace them tomorrow. He gets nothing."

No confrontation ever came. I wouldn't have minded if it had. Because I had unlocked something: Over the course of the evening, I had stopped myself from thinking about going back and getting that dressing gown cord sorted, I had stopped thinking about how much I hated myself and how much I hated my family. I had only thought about how spectacular the special effects were in The Last Starfighter (so sue me, it was the very early 1990s!) and how much I loved the musical score (and *Catherine Mary Stewart* too!). I got lost in the colour and the spectacle of Flash Gordon, sucked in completely with the world John Carpenter built inside of Escape From New York and how crazy and savage it all felt. I laughed at the shtick in Running Scared and loved the big shoot-out ending whilst my jaw-dropped at the still impressive car chase Peter Hyams executed and I walked round for the house for days singing Michael McDonald's 'Sweet Freedom'. (In moments of low mood even to this day, 'Sweet Freedom' is a song I use as a really useful tool to help me remember how far I've come and that I can 'get out' of these so-called "dark places" emotionally and mentally.)

Suddenly it became apparent to me that I had found my 'escape' route just by pressing play on or sitting down in front of a film.

In the same way that I felt so incredibly *seen* the first time I read Roald Dahl's Matilda, I realised that like the protagonist in that novel I could temporarily escape from the life I didn't like being part of - but using films instead of books.

I could stop myself thinking about the worst aspects of what was going on in my day to day life or with my family simply by giving myself over to Kevin Costner bicycle-racing dramas or Rocky sequels, or fantasies involving a man with rocket packs fighting the Nazis, a young farm boy teaming up with a vengeance-obsessed swordsman and a giant to rescue Princess Buttercup or Kurt Russell doing whatever you want to try and explain was going down in the magnificent Big Trouble In Little China.

For the first time, at just fourteen years of age, I felt I had unlocked some sort of *power*: I could travel emotionally away from my troubles and the abuse in my life... using films.

Mental Health, Movies and Me - Part 2

Film became my crutch. In *all* ways. The more I traversed through adolescence the more my parents told me how I was dissatisfactory to them. The more they did that the more I escaped into films. The more I did that the more I would get smacked around or criticised. There never seemed to be an escape from disappointing them and being physically abused. Once I hit my teenage years the comparisons against my elder sister became constant and unrelenting. Even at the point that I excelled over her in my academic qualifications the achievement would have to be diminished down with the "explanation" that I had apparently taken 'easier' GCSEs and/or A-levels. When I passed my driving test first time against her multiple attempts it was because they'd allegedly "lowered the standards" since she did it. It was never-ending.

It was also becoming apparent that there was a great disparity in the care and attention my parents would afford one child over another.

My sister could sit and regale my parents with her travails and outrages, and they would hang on her every word. The opposite was true of me. I was just starting that awkward journey through puberty and adolescence, which is uncomfortable enough as is and at the same time my parents would frequently remind me that I was an irritant.

At the point my self-value and confidence needed to be developing I was being informed daily that I should have no confidence in my value because I "didn't click easily" with people or that I had "silly interests".

On the rare occasions I would venture out to socialise my mother would make me stand at the bottom of the stairs whilst she stood a few steps up to match my height and she would count the spots on my face, which in turn made me self-conscious about people looking at me.

Sometimes I would just head back upstairs and hide away in my room, too worried about going out and having people see my face. I developed this fear that turned into a real belief that if I got too close to a girl and tried to talk to her spots on my face would explode and shoot 'matter' on to hers and I would be a laughingstock. I'd simply pull the blinds closed, pull out another video of some b-movie I had illicitly taped off BBC2's Moviedrome series and... escape from my thoughts!

My parents' fickle disinterest in me could be exemplified by how little concern they had when I was out the house for hours on end. As an adult I once asked my mother whether she was ever worried where I was when I disappeared for eight to ten hours at a time on a Saturday at such a young age. I was informed by her that they didn't care, they were just happy that I was "out from underneath [them]".

In the immediate aftermath of that 'awakening' over Christmas, I fell into a routine every Saturday; I'd get up and ride my bike into the shopping centre on the edge of my estate, I'd visit the local library there and read graphic novels, hire out books and then ride down to the local video shop where I'd spend easily an hour pouring over blurbs and poster art. The shop owners became so friendly with me that they eventually gave me a 'junior' card and let me rent anything that was a 'U' or 'PG' certificate. Very occasionally they'd let me slip a '15' out of the store – which is how I got my first experience of Big Trouble In Little China, so obsessed with the poster art for that film was I. Watching that film for the first time blew my fragile little mind. Fourteen years of age is probably the *perfect age* to experience that film and the insanity it offers.

I'd hire a couple of titles out – frequently it would be the likes of American Flyers or BMX Bandits, The Goonies and what not, again and again – then cross over to the newsagents and buy myself some sweets for the viewing experience.

As my age crept up, I started to take the metro to the local multiplex of an afternoon. My parents didn't care where I was as long as I was back home by no later than five thirty so they could feed me then get ready to go out for the evening together. They never asked where I'd been or who I'd been with. They always presumed I'd been "playing out" but I often didn't have anyone to play out with.

I didn't have many friends growing up and I didn't make them easily. I wasn't confident enough to interact with people my own age because I had a perpetual fear that they would make fun of me the way my own family did. As I got a little bit older in my teenage years, I would mask my lack of confidence with a faked zany 'bluster' to make other kids think I was more than what I considered myself to be. They could see through it. Often people would find me good company or funny in small doses then very quickly tire of my try-hard mentality and cast me aside. This was something that continued for most of my life too.

Even at a young age I was taking the criticisms my parents bestowed upon me and looking at the confidence and ease of my classmates and I was realising that I didn't have the sort of 'personality' that lent itself to people being able to find me tolerable at the most basic level - at least for more than a couple of hours at a time anyway. I'd try to make friends but the type of person I am seemingly lent itself to being easily used and/or quickly put down.

It wasn't always like this though.

When I was a child there was a boy who saw something in me that others did not and could not.

He was in my class and lived close by my grandparents, where I spent most of my time in school holidays and weekends.

We were bonded by our loneliness amidst a sea of heads at school as much as our shared sense of humour. Even at a young age I came to appreciate this friend for simply liking *me* and we quickly became inseparable.

On the last day of school, with a vast and limitless summer ahead of us before separate high schools would provide an inevitable divide, we had an argument. A silly, stupid, nothing argument that degenerated into shoving and me accidentally banging his head off a bathroom wall during lunchbreak by mistake. We left school that day with our friendship impacted and the first week of the summer holiday's heavily damaged by him not being by my side in it.

And on the very night that I finally decided I didn't want this to continue any longer... that the very next morning I would pick up the phone and ask him if he wanted to go ride bikes in the dene... he died.

An asthma attack. A fuckin *asthma attack.*

He died believing that I was not his friend and that devastated me. It still does. Thirty-something years later, I think about Neil at least once a week. I see clips of talent show magicians and *know* that'd have been him. I've tried all my life to replicate a friendship like it and I've never succeeded. (Even in my late teens when I met someone who I clicked with on every level and adored equal to my own grandparents, I let the friendship implode over something stupid because I had such low self-esteem at that time, I couldn't bring myself to stand up against a lie told to this friend about me that decimated our relationship.)

But can we ever generate that closeness in adulthood towards someone like we could as children when we were free of responsibility and bonded by limitless possibility?

Remember how earlier we looked at self-esteem and how it is needed not just to make us feel like we are good enough but also to be able to move past mistakes we have made and to proportionately hold ourselves to account fairly?

I've frequently wondered what my life would've been like if Neil had still been in it, telling myself over and over that this would've been one of the rare pre-teen childhood friendships that lasted.

I miss him and would give anything to be able to deliver the apology to him that he deserved then and is still owed now because I still have trouble forgiving myself over him leaving this earth thinking there was a time when we weren't friends.

The distance in my relationship with my parents during my teenage years widened in direct correlation to how their relationship with my sister tightened, eventually manifesting itself in them booking a family holiday for the three of them and telling me that my sister hadn't wanted me to go because I was "annoying", with my father adding on the end "We just presumed you'd want to hang out with your grandma and grandad?"

They went off to some Spanish resort for two weeks and I rocked up on my grandparent's doorstep with a hold-all full of clothes and a box full of videotapes. That first night we tucked into my grandma's sausage and egg butties and watched Major League together. My grandma wanted to turn it off because it was "too rude". I convinced her to see it through because it had a happy ending. By the time the climax occurred my grandma cheered at the TV. I smile remembering this. I recall turning to her and saying "Thanks for this. You know? Putting me up?" She smiled back and said, "Well where else were you going to go, you silly sod!"

That night I lay in bed in my grandparents' spare room and my grandfather came into the room, sat on the edge of the bed, and stared at his lap. He was not an emotional man. He didn't speak his feelings and you generally measured his happiness by the pat he'd bestow upon your leg or shoulder if you'd done something good. On this night though, whilst still staring down at his lap he simply said, "You know you are loved, don't you?" I slowly nodded my head. He nodded too then left.

We never spoke any further on this.

There was no expansion from him regarding it. That was it. I often think about what he must have been thinking at that time or what he was seeing from his own perspective that made him feel he needed to say that. I think about it now as an adult with two children myself and I'm thankful.

By the time I was sixteen years of age I was a mess. I was starting to want relationships with girls and had no understanding whatsoever as to how to talk to them, with so much of my formative years having hidden away in my bedroom too terrified to go out because of the 'physical monstrousness' I was led to believe I possessed. I wanted to be more confident yet felt I had nothing to offer anyone. I felt like if I just did what my parents asked of me then this would make them love and respect me equal to my sister and then, bam, everything would be *alright*. Or something.

This 'thirst' to be accepted by anyone, everyone or someone led me to be a very easy target for bullies and my teenage years saw me suffer some horrendous acts of violence from people I was trying to befriend with an overzealousness that made them hungrier to reject me as 'weird'.

I was stabbed repeatedly with compasses in the back until the blood flowed into my underpants. (The ones used for drawing perfect circles. Not the ones for showing you directions. I wouldn't normally stop proceedings to point this out, but I once told this to a therapist who then spent several sessions thereafter presuming it was the latter so... God, imagine the blunt force trauma you'd sustain from getting stabbed with one of *those* compasses?) I would come home in agony, get told off by my parents for ruining school shirts and then interrogated as to why I was making people behave like this towards me.

I was once held down by each limb so someone could repeatedly try out elbow drops and high plummeting wrestling moves on my face.

This resulted in me being required to be picked up unconscious where I'd been left in the school yard and carried into the nurses' office.

I recall my parents being summoned to school to pick me up and encouraged thereafter to go get me checked out at hospital, and on that occasion an English teacher who had great affection for me grabbed my father by the arm and said to him in my presence "You've got to get him out of this school or they're going to keep going until they kill him. Don't you understand?" I remember this vividly.

I had zero self-esteem and a feeling that I was not worthy of belonging anywhere by the time I left my teens and entered the world of work. I just had this overwhelming need to please people and for someone or anyone to tell me that I was good and that I had something to offer. I'd already been faced with the stark reality that university was not going to be the 'cushy number' for me that it was for my sister; my parents hadn't saved for me like they had for her because they told me they never expected me to "lean that way, academically". I begged my parents but because I wanted to do a degree in something film or writing related and not what they wanted me to do they told me they wouldn't assist outside of giving me a thousand pounds. The rest I would need to find myself. I tried accessing grants, bursaries, you name it. My parents earned too much for me to get the financial assistance I needed. My grandmother offered to help. My dad blocked her. I simply couldn't afford to go.

I left school and joined the military instead simply because I saw it offering a myriad of benefits; all of my favourite writers growing up had served in the military in one way or another at some point and written memoirs about it *and* it would get me away from my family and force me to start developing some confidence in myself, what I had to offer and the like. It was one of the biggest mistakes I made in my life and, with both of my grandfather's having died by this point, it fell on my grandmother to try and talk me out of it. I ignored her and I regret that to this very day.

Forget the marketing campaigns about how the army / navy / air force can "make a man" out of you and help build confidence, self-esteem whilst broadening your horizons.

Blah, blah. Blah and blah.

It's nonsense.

The military environment, it goes without saying, is an absolute 'alpha' one that needs fed, and it feeds on the weak, the underconfident and all those suckers who bought the bullshit the marketing campaigns and the school talks on careers' day spoon out.

Once again, I was ruthlessly bullied but this time the bullying was dialled up a whole other notch because there isn't any teacher stepping in or parent coming to pull you apart. The figures of authority aren't looking to stop it. They're looking to watch how you react to it, overcome it and so forth.

I would work harder than anyone else in my unit, thinking that's what it would take for them to respect me and accept me, but all this did was make them realise that they could exploit that. It was an experience that followed me through every job thereafter. The only difference with this one is that they trained me to kill, had me do so and then opened the door at the other end for me to fumble out the other side bruised, broken and disturbed in just under a year.

My parents saw my failure at my first attempt at a career as a validation of their criticisms of me throughout my upbringing. And they would frequently tell me so. I started to drink just to be able to get to sleep without thinking about some of the things I'd seen and done in my short tenure within military life. I would bounce from career to career throughout my entire twenties, desperately looking for a place just to rest and be accepted – my life became just a rotating circle of cigarettes and alcohol, eight hours in some job I didn't give a shit about, coming home with a takeaway to a barely furnished flat, sitting watching film after film alone and occasionally venturing into ill-considered relationships with women I was not attracted to, who had 'baggage' or emotional issues and who I was just happy to have display an interest in me.

In every job I could never find that all important 'medium speed'.

I was either fully committed and too keen to the point that I would repulse my colleagues and get exploited by my managers.

Or I would be so indifferent or unenthusiastic about what I was doing that I was quickly managed out of the role and shown the door.

It didn't matter, as long as I could come home and drown it all out in front of films.

It wasn't a life. It was an existence.

Each relationship I entered during this time, if you could call them that, would come with my parents' immediate pressure as to whether this was 'the one' and whether I was finally going to "settle down" and "sort [my] life out". I was a functioning alcoholic with the occasional penchant for heating up knives and drawing them across my skin to give myself a momentary pause from my thoughts. I had zero business being in a relationship with anyone, yet I bounded from one to another. Each taking advantage of me for what money I had or my home.

I didn't care. This was all just stuff that was happening *around* me. If there was beer in the fridge, a full pack of Lucky Strike Lights and a pile of films waiting to be watched then I was "happy". But I clearly wasn't. Because I was self-harming frequently, routinely bursting into tears and on one occasion I attempted suicide (only for it to end up in the most pathetic farce you could possibly muster). I became overly attached to the Sidney Lumet film, The Verdict, because I saw so much of myself in Paul Newman's character of Frank Galvin.

In the film Galvin is an outcast in the legal profession and a full blown alcoholic reduced to drinking out his days and chasing down ambulances for shitty personal injury cases. His best friend and fellow lawyer Mickey Morrissey (Jack Warden) hands him a 'Silver Platter' of a medical malpractice suit with all parties willing to settle out of court, but Galvin sees this as an opportunity to punish the guilty, right wrongs and to restore his standing as a lawyer and he blunders ahead with a full trial regardless.

The film has this great speech in it, written by the once mighty David Mamet, where Galvin sums up the case before the jury.

I used to have the speech memorised. I used to frequently get drunk alone and stand in my living room reciting it between cigarette draws.

In the original draft of this book under its first title there was an excerpt right about here from The Verdict's script of Galvin's big, final court speech. Obviously all I can do now is direct you to YouTube it, or even better to watch the film itself if you've never seen it and observe the speech in its proper context. It's a masterpiece of a film and Paul Newman gives his best ever performance, and that's saying a lot because he was one of the greatest actors there's ever been.

I believed I was Frank Galvin. I believed my shot – my redemption – was coming. But it wasn't. And I would crash hard when I would invest majorly (in a career or an opportunity with a zealousness around righting my own wrongs or finally being seen as worthy in the eyes of my parents) and it would fail.

I would go to see a GP and they'd provide me with pills. And the pills wouldn't work so they'd give me different pills. They didn't work either, but all the side effects did instead. Round and round this façade would go. Interspersed with occasional attempts at therapy which would always either be short-lived in their timeframe before any real effect took place or fruitless because of how little I put into it or how much bullshit I littered the sessions with as I had yet to learn to be honest with myself.

Ten years on from all of this I would end up diagnosed with PTSD (post-traumatic stress disorder) and suddenly things started making sense.

They got a little bit easier too.

Because once you can see your enemy you can fight back against them a lot better.

Here's the most interesting and transformative thing about receiving the PTSD diagnosis...

... and why you'll see I'm not anti-therapy, more all about finding the right type and emotionally investing in it properly...

It was the moment the psychologist revealed my trauma pre-dated my experience(s) in uniformed services that left me so troubled.

I initially braced against the hypothesis. Loads of people grow up having been "slapped around" by their parents or not being "emotionally nurtured" properly. They don't all end up a fuck-up like me. "Did you have trouble sleeping before you went into the military?" the psychologist countered. I nodded. "And did that have to do with your father breaking your nose in your sleep?" I nodded again. "You talk about how if you are woken from sleep by loud noises or too suddenly it can induce severe panic and anxiety, and that this used to happen even as a child – do you see where I am going here?"

That conversation was the first chip away at the robust wall I had put up around myself and my mental health. It was certainly the start of me transforming my relationship with myself, my family and my own emotional wellbeing. But in that regard, we must roll back to what I said in the introduction:

Part of the transformation around my wellbeing came with looking at my esteem issues and the labelling of myself as a 'failure'. Every time I'd take the antidepressants or do the course of therapy or go celibate or stop speaking at work... or just not do the things that I thought annoyed people or brought difficulties upon me... depression would <u>still</u> pop its head back up. With it would come the desire to kill myself and be free of the weight of these wholly negative feelings because I couldn't be 'cured'.

The seismic shift occurred in two forms.

The first was in meeting my wife.

And with my wife came her family and friends.

Through them I saw life differently for the first time – I saw what familial love looked like and positive reinforcement too.

Their accepting of me into their family and my wife choosing to spend the rest of her life with me brought about this thought that I *must* have some value if people like this have a regard, an affection and/or love for me.

One day I referred to myself as a "failure" in the presence of my wife and she replied "You see a failure. I see a survivor."

The second came through me one day asking myself whether these thoughts, feelings, emotions etc weren't things that could be 'cured' but were things I had to learn to live with and keep at bay by looking at life differently as well as treating it differently too. I was stuck in a perpetual circle in which every time a depressive episode, a panic attack or an issue of severe anxiety occurred I would treat it as if it was 'back' and that not being able to 'beat it' was another example of failure that exasperated my negative feelings. Arriving at the point of looking differently at my mental health, challenging it and exploring it was my 'John McClane' moment of realising that the support outside of Nakatomi Plaza wasn't going to do much unless I rose to face the challenge inside at the same time too.

I asked myself whether these mental health issues could simply be *in* us, like negative personality quirks – we can be greedy, we can all be selfish, we can be moody, etc etc. but part of how we mature is in recognising that in ourselves and minimising those qualities as best we can. The foibles in our personality, good and bad, make us who we are. What if our mental health is the same? It's a part of all of us and part of what makes us who we are. We're all susceptible to it whether that's through grief, stress, loneliness and so forth but it is how we *manage* it rather than *cure* it. That was the day I defined my own depression as a 'black cloud' that is always up there, above me and that I needed to find ways to stay one step ahead of it.

I did this by starting to have a more honest, internal dialogue with myself around the "important stuff" like antidepressants and therapy.

I started to look at the relationships both around me and the ones I have mentally and emotionally with myself in terms of catastrophising and problem solving.

These things alone helped formulate a difference in how I set goals for myself and how I managed stress, which in turn seeped into how and why I exercised or where I drew joy from. Most interestingly, it changed my relationship with films from being one where they were a crutch I leant too dependently upon to one where they became a useful tool I could draw emotional use from.

I have spent these last two chapters laying all my personal 'stuff' out for you to see so that you'd reach this far in the book... before we've even really got to the 'meat'... and you'd ask yourself how on earth I could have endured the upbringing I had, seen traumatic things, been so crippled with dark depressive episodes that I've attempted suicide and self-harm and still be alive to talk about.

And these are only the things I'm willing to share publicly, think about *that*.

My answer to that lies in the above paragraph.

The things I did and still do now, daily in fact, worked and work for me, and I honestly think they can work for you too.

I'm legally prevented from saying '*will* work', apparently.

Sorry.

"I Feel Seen" #1

WELCOME TO THE DOLLHOUSE

Films to me are like what photographs are to most people – you look at a photograph and think "Oh, I remember that holiday. That was the time..." or "I remember that lad. God, I've not spoken to them in ages!" I'm like that with films. I look at The Rocketeer and I'm reminded of kissing a girl for the first time. I watch North Shore and I'm taken straight back to Sunday afternoons at my grandparents' house. I also believe strongly that films are a great 'unifier'.

I'm not just talking about the communal experience of sitting together inside of a cinema and laughing on mass at a comedy or jumping in unison at a horror film. I am talking about how they can make us feel a little less alone in this world. We see our problems represented up on screen and suddenly said problems don't feel so singular and specific; straight away, there, and then, we've taken a little bit of the weight out of them.

The first time I ever recall taking note of this and having it make an impact on me I was a few weeks away from my sixteenth birthday:

My parents' weekends were spent 'pottering' before heading off to the pub for the evening together.

My dad's entire Saturday was built around going to the betting shop then coming home and watching racing events on TV all afternoon.

My mum's was spent obsessively tidying the house around him.

I would disappear out of the door first thing on a Saturday and head to the local multiplex where I'd spend the day watching one or two films.

Sometimes with friends that I temporarily had at the time but mostly on my own.

On this Saturday I'd fled the house in tears because of an argument with my mum over a coat.

You see, for the longest time I was obsessed with this coat in the window of a cheap leather store on the local high street. It was black suede with old Native American pattern work stitched across the main torso and tassels – yes, fuckin *tassels* – hanging off the shoulders.

I can look at it in my minds' eye now and recognise that it was truly hideous but back then I *loved* it and coveted it badly.

I'd saved up my pocket money, I'd done extra chores, I cut down on my video rentals and within two months I had accrued enough money to buy this jacket and I was so excited. My mother drove me to the shop to buy it, took one look at it and refused outright to do so. She said it was "vile" and there was no way I would be seen in it. I argued that it was my earned money, and I should be allowed to spend it on what I like. She disagreed. I broke my heart to my grandparents that weekend over this and they agreed there and then to buy it for me as an early present for my upcoming sixteenth birthday. Which they did. And which my mum monumentally lost her shit instantly over – tearing the jacket and throwing it in the bin immediately in front of my grandma and grandad. (Both she and my father didn't speak to my grandparents for over a year because of this jacket incident.)

I left the house the morning after 'jacket-gate' and went up to the city centre, changing my usual routine from the local multiplex to the art-house cinema a mile or so over the bridge.

I was looking for somewhere that would be showing the latest John Carpenter film, a director I'd become obsessed with (the film in question that year was his disastrous remake of Village of the Damned), and I was convinced seeing as my usual cinema didn't have it on the more '*arty*' place might.

Of course, they didn't but what they did have starting momentarily was a film I'd never heard of called Welcome To The Dollhouse.

How quaint a time it was to grow up not having the internet and getting exhausted by a film before it's even been released.

I looked at the poster.

It said it was a "hilarious black comedy".

"A comedy? I could do with being cheered up!" I naively thought. I theorised I could go see this and then squeeze in more of a blockbuster type deal afterwards back over the road.

The film played out before me, and my jaw dropped.

It wasn't just that it was so off-kilter and tonally quite unlike anything I'd seen before, and I considered myself a wide-ranging film nut even at that age. It wasn't that it had all the rough-hewn charm of a micro-budgeted indie movie smack-bang in the middle of the independent cinema boom of the 1990s.

It was that it felt so... so... *autobiographical* it made me uncomfortable. I remember looking around the cinema in certain moments, bewildered and confused, wondering whether I was victim of some hidden camera stunt on a TV show I wasn't yet aware of.

Todd Solondz' film is a coming-of-age dark comedy – and I mean *dark*; with three A's in the middle, italicised and boldened.

You can probably get a measure as to how dark by the fact that its original title was Faggots & Retards.

It tells the story of a deeply unpopular twelve year old girl called Dawn Wiener who lives as the middle child with her more popular siblings and her two wildly disinterested parents who think Dawn is a detriment and an embarrassment to the family.

The film follows Dawn through her family and scholastic life - a life she is very visibly physically uncomfortable within - as she's viciously bullied and abused yet constantly found living in hope of better days whilst lying to herself that she is better regarded than she is.

I came out of the art house cinema and almost staggered from the alleyway it was based in.

I kept thinking about the film over and over.

There were lines of dialogue in that film that were *actual* things my own parents had said to me.

Dawn Wiener:
"I was fighting back!"

Mrs Wiener:
"Who told you to fight back?"

There were hurtful terms and painful actions carried out against Dawn at school that had quite literally happened to me. How was this possible?

I did something I had never done before on a visit to the cinema. I turned back round, went up to the poster to scribble down on the back of my metro ticket the name 'Todd Solondz' then I went back into the cinema and watched the film again on its next showing.

My shock turned to a big, broad grin as I suddenly realised that these things I was experiencing from my family and at school weren't just happening to me.

They were happening to other people too.

All over the world in fact.

Some were writing stories about it that became films. That was something that could *happen*? My mind was racing!

I had to learn about this Todd Solondz fella though. Did he know me? Is that what this was?

Yeah, fifteen year old me was walking away from this situation believing I'd been the victim of a theft of my life-rights. I had to know more about him and in the mid 1990s that took fucking *time*, let me tell you.

We were a pre-internet age.

You couldn't just abuse the shit out of someone by typing a sentence and pressing send on social media.

You had to get the hell up, seek them out and say it to their face.

And in that same breath, if you wanted to learn more about a movie star or a director you had to trawl through film almanacs and textbooks or look through film magazines.

That's what I had to do to learn about Solondz.

He didn't stand out to me as being an exceptional man nor a man who could in some ways have heard about me or my life and stole it wholesale. He was simply an ex teacher of English to Russian immigrants in New York City who wrote screenplays in his spare time and made short films. Welcome To The Dollhouse was what he had broken through with.

I felt a deep, important connection with a man I'd never met. I felt less lonely and suddenly a little bit empowered because Dawn Wiener had met each abusive challenge with an unwavering reaction of awkward positivity, I could try doing that too. I'd never, ever talked to anyone or felt close enough to anyone to talk about my life at home and how my parents hurt me or bullied me. Yet somehow, I felt I had been heard without speaking through this film.

Films unexpectedly gained more power and influence in my life that day. It wouldn't be the first time a film had come along that made an impact upon me and helped me emotionally. We'll look at some more a little later. It would be decades later though before I learnt how to harness that power and influence to positive effect properly.

Part Two

'Magic Pills':
Antidepressants and You

I am not *anti* anti-depressants. And that's not what this chapter is going to be about. I know many people that are using them now, long-term. I know people who have utilised them on a short-term basis. They would describe positive experiences and positive outcomes from doing so. Equally, I have had friends who've taken them and had terrible experiences from the side-effects or continue to pop them daily now because it is innately built into their morning routine, yet they have never once yielded anything positive from taking them and no GP has ever wound them down off them.

Antidepressants simply don't work for *all* people. And I think a lot of the time our relationship to them is one moulded by severely unrealistic expectations – that they're a 'magic pill' that we take and then we feel happy, and now everything is alright because we're happy. It's not like that. Your success in finding one that works for you and carries a benefit is absolutely the same as all other facets of support around mental health; the more honest you are with the medical professional and yourself the more beneficial the result is.

It took me the longest time to realise this and to understand it properly and even then, I've still yet to find an antidepressant that works for me in even the most mildly impactive form.

You can't just role up into a GP surgery, having googled "strongest and most effective antidepressant", quickly study the screenshot you took of the search results and ask for the finest Citalopram, Sertraline, Escitalopram or Paroxetine in all the land.

They'll be onto you damn quick that you're phoning this whole thing in. You also must be accepting of the fact most doctors now have a 'start low, raise slowly' policy when it comes to prescribing antidepressants and they are normally always done so as part of what's called combination-treatment, i.e. seeing a counsellor, receiving CBT (cognitive behavioural therapy), etc.

They're not just wanting you to lie at home and pop the pills. They're expecting you to put the work in to get better too – do you see where the John McClane in Die Hard / 'stepping up' analogy is sliding its way into play here?

And that's *difficult*. I know. I've been there at both ends of the scale – when you can't be fucked with any of that and you just want the "magic pill" but also when you commit to attending the appointments, bearing your soul, filling in the silly worksheets that have outdated clipart on them and you get no return from your effort.

Let's have a go at breaking the whole antidepressants thing down into the most crayon-thick layman's terms possible and see if you learn anything about them in some capacity that helps explain why things might not have worked for you in the past or educate you more going forward so that you can make decisions about what to take or even whether to take them.

So... yeah... we all know that antidepressant medications are a popular and encouraged option for treating mental health issues such as depression, anxiety and the like, right? Next slide? *Okay*.

There are different antidepressants that work differently with the brain and are therefore better at dealing with one area of mental health than another. They're split into 'families', of sorts. Like the Montagues and the Capulets, if you're classy. Or the Butchers and the Mitchells if you're not. Though they're not at war with each other. They probably don't even *know* of each other. You know what? This analogy needs work. Let's move on.

Whilst some 'families' of antidepressants are better for treating certain conditions and symptoms than others, nearly all of them bar none come with side effects that exist on a sliding scale of impact. That's where your own honest assessment of self and the response to taking antidepressants is important because the dialogue you have with your GP around dosage increases, coming off them etc is wholly relative to what positive you're seeing in your mood and outlook versus the impact that you're suffering in other ways. (We'll cover that more in a moment.)

Everybody's reaction to antidepressants is individual in much the same way everyone's experience of side effects is frequently singular to themselves. I've taken antidepressants that have left me constipated and unable to stay awake. I have had a friend take the same medication at the exact same dosage and they've poo'd for days like someone has broken the dam in the film Hard Rain. I've taken tablets that have given me zero side effect and zero benefit yet I've known people who have taken the same medication and been hit with every side effect going whilst getting minimal uptick from doing so, making it very hard to justify staying on them long term as had been advised.

The aforementioned 'families' themselves are:

- SSRIs - Selective serotonin reuptake inhibitors
- SNRIs - Serotonin-norepinephrine reuptake inhibitors
- TCAs - Tricyclic antidepressants
- And MAOIs - Monoamine oxidase inhibitors

Worry not, there's not going to be a quiz in which you're expected to remember your norepinephrine from your oxidase. We'll break them down together, nickname them so they're easier to associate and look at what they do and what negatives they offer up in return.

SSRIs are the popular antidepressant of choice for treating the likes of anxiety disorders, PTSD, OCD, hot flashes, and panic:

There's a 'trouble spot' (i.e. the brain) and the military (your GP) knows who to call to "get the job done" (in sorting out your serotonin). We'll call SSRIs **'John Rambos'**. Low levels of serotonin are thought to play a big role in depression. It is one type of a neurotransmitter that affects your mood. Usually when your brain releases serotonin a lot of it is used to communicate with other cells, whilst some goes back into the cell that released it. 'John Rambos' decrease the amount of serotonin that goes to other cells and leaves more available in your brain.

Types of 'John Rambos' you can get are Celexa (branded as citalopram), Lexapro (escitalopram), good ol' Prozac (which is a brand of fluoxetine) and Zoloft (sertraline). The side effects of taking them however can include headaches, nausea, trouble sleeping, dizziness, diarrhea, weakness, fatigue, increased anxiety, upset stomach, dry mouth, increased appetite (leading to weight gain) and issues of low sex drive and erectile dysfunction or ejaculation problems in men. 'John Rambos' are known for causing sexual side effects more than other antidepressants.

I have had experience of taking sertraline and I suffered greatly with no real positive outcome other than initially feeling less panicked. This wore off very quickly though and what I was left with was sometimes crippling headaches I was told would fade and didn't, diarrhea, a constant feeling of fatigue and an increase in weight because I was never not hungry.

The Rambo movies were successful enough and such was Sylvester Stallone and Arnold Schwarzenegger's rivalry in the 1980s that the latter purposefully went out of his way to make sure he had his own 'Rambo'. This was in the form of the movie Commando where he played Colonel John Matrix. He's ostensibly Rambo but... you know... *different*. Because Matrix has a daughter and he's kicking arse for her, not for his country. Otherwise, yeah Commando offers up a whole lot of the same 'sauce' as Rambo.

With that in mind, if your 'John Rambos' aren't doing it or your GP wants to consider an alternative route, there's your **'Colonel Matrix'** antidepressants.

That's what SNRIs ostensibly are. They work the same way as 'John Rambos', only they're trying to take on neurotransmitters like norepinephrine as well as serotonin because... well... they're ballsy like that, I guess.

Some people I have spoken with say a course of 'Colonel Matrix' is better than 'John Rambos' for that reason. I don't know enough from experience in ingesting them to be able to agree or disagree there. I do know however that Arnold Schwarzenegger's Commando is better than all the Rambo sequels combined (but not First Blood).

'Colonel Matrix' medication can be used to treat depression and depression-related issues, but they are also used to treat fibromyalgia and nerve damage resultant from diabetes. The side effects from taking them are really the same as 'John Rambos' with profuse sweating and raised blood pressure getting added to the list, but the difference is most reports seem to indicate that 'Colonel Matrix' can cause more weight *loss* in people than weight *gain* though the latter is still a possibility. Known medications under the 'Colonel Matrix' banner would be things like desvenlafaxine, duloxetine, levomilnacipran and venlafaxine.

Do you remember an 'old' (God, how depressing to regard a film made in 2000 as "old") Clint Eastwood film called Space Cowboys? It starred Clint Eastwood, Tommy Lee Jones, Donald Sutherland and James Garner (one of my favourite actors) as aged, retired ex test pilots who are called upon by NASA to re-train and go into space as pensioners and fix a satellite issue that only they can do. Well, TCA's are '**The Space Cowboys**'.

They're a much older type of antidepressant, which like 'Colonel Matrix', help to increase levels of norepinephrine and serotonin in your brain.

But where they're different is they also decrease the effects of another neurotransmitter called acetylcholine and in doing so they risk increasing side effects.

Yup, that's an increase in headaches, nausea, trouble sleeping, dizziness, diarrhea, weakness, fatigue, increased anxiety, upset stomach, dry mouth, weight gain and sexual side effects; so nowadays they are only generally used when 'John Rambos' and 'Colonel Matrix' aren't working well for you and have been properly and sufficiently explored across a range of types and dosages.

'The Space Cowboys' come with the same side effects as 'John Rambos' and 'Colonel Matrix' but often more *frequently* and more *severely*, alongside potentially dangerous effects like abnormal heart rate or arrhythmia, high blood pressure and sudden blood pressure drops when standing up. The types of 'Space Cowboys' known the most are the likes doxepin, imipramine, nortriptyline, amitriptyline, clomipramine and desipramine.

I have taken a course of amitriptyline and it did wonders in terms of improving my sleep because it had me zonked or feeling that way a lot of the time; getting more sleep in turn helped me be able to combat more of the day to day troubles I was facing but they didn't do anything for my overall mood and in the long-term I knew that this level of sleepiness couldn't be sustained alongside full time work. My weight also crept up too and I noticed an impact upon the quality of sex I was having with my partner at the time too.

Finally, within our breakdown, there's the MAOIs.

You know how you had that one friend who used to always get drunk too quickly on nights out, get in bother and inevitably say something offensive but you kind of had to stick with him because he was the only single one amongst you and you saw benefit in having his place to crash back at and 'keep the party going' once the pubs and clubs had closed...

... but then you got older and you got wiser, and more mature in realising that as your priorities and perspectives in life shifted so too did any interest in maintaining a friendship with the fist-throwing, easily drunk racist friend in your group just because he had a 'crash pad'? Especially seeing as you don't really go out that much anymore.

Well, the MAOIs are **'The Jim Coopers'**. (Yeah, my friend within this analogy *was* named Jim Cooper. It'll not get past 'legal' for the final publishable draft. Don't worry.) They're not really fit for purpose as an antidepressant, some doctors occasionally still lean on them though in an 'if all else fails' situation because they break down certain neurotransmitters and by doing so, they can increase your levels of serotonin, norepinephrine, and dopamine. Really though, they're mostly forgotten about as an antidepressant within the medical circles I spoke with for this book. 'The Jim Coopers' now work more towards assisting in the treatment of Parkinson's disease than depression.

That's the main 'lot'. I could go on. But I won't. I mean, do you really want to be hearing in-depth shit about medicines and medications from someone who's strongest tie to the medical profession is that I once got to do a telephone interview with Andy Garcia and I told him I was a big fan of Desperate Measures (his ostensible 'Die Hard in a hospital' film with Michael Keaton from 1998 that mostly sank without a trace) and he replied "You liked that movie, huh?" and then there was a huge long awkward silence – because, between you and me, I think *he* didn't.

Anyway, let me just quickly mention that outside of 'John Rambos', 'Colonel Matrix', 'The Space Cowboys' and 'The Jim Coopers' there's also atypical antidepressants – or, you know, 'rogue agents' – which don't fit into the "families" made up of 'John Rambos', 'Colonel Matrix, etc. etc.

There's bupropion (which concentrates on dopamine increases rather than targeting doesn't serotonin) and mirtazapine (which if we had time I'd call 'The Bad Bitch' and go into more detail because she's known as a serotonin antagonist and she goes after the norepinephrine, serotonin <u>and</u> dopamine in your brain in a different way than other antidepressants) but, you know, I can see your eyes glazing over and I don't want to lose you so... we'll move on.

As a quick aside, I did once ask a GP to be put on a course of mirtazapine after starting to take a more detailed interest in the medications I was on, their impact, what worked and what didn't etc. etc.

She refused.

I asked why.

She said "I don't prescribe by request. I'm a doctor. Not a DJ."

Five years later I saw an article in the newspaper that she'd been struck off the medical register over a proven allegation of negligence. She's now a wedding DJ.

No, I'm joking. About the DJ thing, not getting struck off. Wouldn't it be brilliant if she *was* a DJ now though? I don't know what she is.

But I'm glad she's not a GP anymore.

The bottom line is that there's a whole heap of medication out there that can work, can work in combination with other medications, cannot prove effective or can deliver side effects impactive enough that the bad outweighs the good. The whole antidepressant thing is a *journey*, and the easier, more effective journey occurs when you're honest with yourself and more importantly your GP or medical support about first your symptoms and then your experience(s) whilst taking any antidepressants.

I learnt this the hard way.

Throughout my twenties I was embarrassed to talk about my thoughts and feelings. Certainly with a doctor. Even more so with a doctor who was my long-time family GP and knew my parents and grandparents very well.

I frequently undersold both the depth of my negative feeling(s) and more pertinently the amount of alcohol I was consuming to get through the day (alcohol and antidepressants are not good bedfellows – at all!).

Symptoms of depression differ per person and at different intensity levels and there may be one antidepressant that is better at tackling a certain type of symptom than another. If you know family members (specifically blood relatives) that have suffered from depression and had success with one type of antidepressant this is also worth discussing with your GP because there is a possibility it might work for you too.

I offered up no tangible detail initially when discussing my mental health with GPs. I just mumbled the same shit about "not getting enjoyment out of anything anymore" and "not being able to sleep". They'd give me antidepressants. I'd take them then attend a review with the doctor a couple of months later. There'd be no change in my mood, just weight gain or headaches or constant nausea. They'd up the dosage. The mood would stay the same, the side effects wouldn't abate. I'd then give up on them in a reckless and uncontrolled manner.

Repeat ad nauseum.

I got better – and more *responsible* – when it comes to antidepressants the older I got and the more I have started to try to take back some modicum of control over my mental health experience. I've now gotten to a point where I feel confident that antidepressants don't work for me. I really wish they did but once I moved away from the unrealistic 'magic pill' expectation we discussed earlier and once I started to really focus in on my journey and experience with them, it become apparent that they simply did not and it was no longer sensible of me to keep taking a medication that only provided me with too many constant negatives (headaches, diarrhea, fatigue, dry mouth, weight gain) against any tangible positive.

To assess your relationship with antidepressants is an easy one. Firstly, you need to be conscientious and realistic with the medication you're taking to give it a fair old shake at doing its job. I have what I call 'The Magnificent Seven Golden Rules' in this regard. They are as follows and you need to adhere to *all* of them:

1. **Be patient:**

Some people see a change develop within a couple of weeks but the average person, certainly among friends and people I spoke to for this book, don't start to see an improvement until around four to six weeks. It can take up to eight weeks for the 'ratio' to settle down in terms of the positive improvement versus the adverse side effects. No one sees a magical mood shift within a matter of days. Give the medication a chance. Whilst waiting to give it a chance, slowly introduce the other strategies I talk about later in the book around adjustments in your life that can help.

2. **Knock off the alcohol and drugs:**

There is no remedy to depression at the bottom of a bottle. I should know. I've looked down most. Alcohol makes depression worse. Recreational drugs temporarily numb, they don't permanently eradicate. Both consumed in combination with antidepressants can make you stop or slow down the effect of the medication, make you ill and prove fatal if you're not careful. A hard stop on usage of drink and drugs would obviously be preferable but that's potentially unrealistic for some people. Certainly try to cut down and eventually cut out both over the first week to two weeks of taking your antidepressants.

3. **Embrace Combination Therapy:**

Therapy on its own is not as effective as talking therapy (known as 'psychotherapy' but generally not referred to that in the public domain so much anymore because of the whole 'psycho' bit in the name.) when applied alongside a course of antidepressants. If your GP offers to get you registered for therapy alongside taking your tablets, absolutely take them up on the offer. We'll talk about therapy more in the next chapter.

4. **Take your medication properly:**

Get into a system / habit of taking your medication at the same time every day and take it in harmony with its predominant effects. What I mean by this if you're taking an antidepressant which can make you drowsy and is intended to help you sleep better, you obviously take it last thing at night. If you're expected to take it before food or with food, do it. Don't skip tablets and if you forget to take one don't double up the next day or whatever. Be responsible and find a system that works for you. (For me personally, when I was taking antidepressants that were a sleep aid, I kept them by the side of the bed and took them last thing at night. When I was required to take them first thing in the morning I had them out on the kitchen bench next to things I knew I would need to use to make breakfast.)

5. **Monitor the positive effects:**

Make sure you're taking stock of when and how the medication is taking effect on you, but also if it is not. You will need to do this to have a responsible and honest dialogue with your GP or clinician. You don't need to keep any sort of detailed diary. I'll show you in a minute what worked for me, and you can try that.

6. **Monitor the negative effects:**

As we've discussed, many antidepressants cause side effects that can improve with time. Some don't. It is important, I've found, to make a brief record of what side effects occur or what changes in your physical self have occurred, when and how long they have lasted for. Most side effects decrease and disappear as your body adjusts to the antidepressant. Again though, some don't. (I found that the headaches and nausea can often go with time. The fatigue and the constant hunger never seemed to. But again, everyone is different.) You don't need to go into humongous amounts of detail. I'll show you the method I used.

7. **Never stop taking an antidepressant 'cold' / without talking to your doctor:**

Have you ever been in that relationship where it just isn't working and you still feel it's 'early days' enough for you to get out of it without any significant damage to either of you so you just call it a day and move on... and they turn full blown stalker on you, keying your car, calling you umpteen times a day and what not? We've all seen the film Fatal Attraction, am I right? Well, some antidepressants are the medicinal equivalent of that if you just cut them dead. The withdrawal symptoms can be significant, and your depression or mental health issue can swing back almost immediately and worsened. That's why it is important to withdraw or taper off responsibly and under the guidance of your GP. Or before you know it your proverbial bunny is boiling in the pan.

With regards to 'rules' five and six, you don't need to over-complicate it at all. When it comes to the latter, I created a very simple table like the one below (I made mine in the note-pad of my phone so it was always handy) and I simply wrote down the side effect or the issue I was experiencing since starting the tablets, when it started and when it ended (if it ended, for that matter):

Name of Medication	Side Effect	Date Started	Date Ended
Amitriptyline	Headaches	1st February 2024	9th February 2024
	Fatigue	1st February 2024	Ongoing
	Weight Gain	1st February 2024	Ongoing

Then when it came to the former, i.e. the positive impacts or changes, I created a scale for measuring which ran from 1 to 5. The bottom of the scale represented 'No Change'. The top? 'Total Change'. It looked like this:

1. No Change
2. Minor Changes in some areas.
3. Noticeable Difference.
4. Significant Change
5. Total Change

... and then, once again, I created a little form on my phone that I could access daily. It was laid out to represent eight to twelve tables. Each table represented one week on the course of this particular antidepressant. At the end of each day, I'd score how I felt based off my scale.

You've got to be prepared to get a record going, an itinerary of sorts. No one else is going to do it for you. Think back to Die Hard as our template, yeah? Even John McClane pulled out a marker pen, used his forearm as a notepad and started keeping track of how many terrorists he had killed, names, etc.

Obviously, the first two or three, maybe even four, tablets should show low numbers or all '1s' for reasons we've discussed around Rule One of 'The Magnificent Seven Golden Rules'. It's where the numbers go after that that's important and will feed into your discussion with your GP about increased dosages, changes in type and so forth. Twelve tables of all '1s' is obviously not good. I've included a hypothetical example of what good could look like below. You look at the list in your 'Side Effects' table and your records in your 'Impact table'. If the list in the first is long but the numbers in the second are low, the reality is that this medication is not working for you. It's no more complicated than that. Here's what a completed one could look like:

Week	Day	Impact	Week	Day	Impact	Week	Day	Impact
	Mon	1		Mon	1		Mon	1
1.	Tues	1	2.	Tues	1	3.	Tues	1
	Wed	1		Wed	1		Wed	1
	Thurs	1		Thurs	1		Thurs	1
	Fri	1		Fri	1		Fri	1
	Sat	1		Sat	1		Sat	1
	Sun	1		Sun	1		Sun	1

Week	Day	Impact	Week	Day	Impact	Week	Day	Impact
	Mon	1		Mon	2		Mon	2
4.	Tues	1	5.	Tues	2	6.	Tues	2
	Wed	1		Wed	2		Wed	2
	Thurs	1		Thurs	2		Thurs	2
	Fri	1		Fri	2		Fri	2
	Sat	1		Sat	2		Sat	3
	Sun	2		Sun	2		Sun	3

Week	Day	Impact	Week	Day	Impact	Week	Day	Impact
	Mon	3		Mon	3		Mon	3
7.	Tues	3	8.	Tues	3	9.	Tues	3
	Wed	3		Wed	3		Wed	3
	Thurs	3		Thurs	3		Thurs	3
	Fri	3		Fri	3		Fri	3
	Sat	3		Sat	3		Sat	3
	Sun	3		Sun	3		Sun	3

Week	Day	Impact	Week	Day	Impact	Week	Day	Impact
10.	Mon	3	11.	Mon	4	12.	Mon	4
	Tues	3		Tues	4		Tues	4
	Wed	3		Wed	4		Wed	4
	Thurs	3		Thurs	4		Thurs	4
	Fri	4		Fri	4		Fri	4
	Sat	4		Sat	4		Sat	4
	Sun	4		Sun	4		Sun	4

Overleaf is an empty one for you to use if you'd like to give it a try. Remember to **be honest** with yourself:

Week	Day	Impact	Week	Day	Impact	Week	Day	Impact
	Mon			Mon			Mon	
1.	Tues		2.	Tues		3.	Tues	
	Wed			Wed			Wed	
	Thurs			Thurs			Thurs	
	Fri			Fri			Fri	
	Sat			Sat			Sat	
	Sun			Sun			Sun	

Week	Day	Impact	Week	Day	Impact	Week	Day	Impact
	Mon			Mon			Mon	
4.	Tues		5.	Tues		6.	Tues	
	Wed			Wed			Wed	
	Thurs			Thurs			Thurs	
	Fri			Fri			Fri	
	Sat			Sat			Sat	
	Sun			Sun			Sun	

Week	Day	Impact	Week	Day	Impact	Week	Day	Impact
	Mon			Mon			Mon	
7.	Tues		8.	Tues		9.	Tues	
	Wed			Wed			Wed	
	Thurs			Thurs			Thurs	
	Fri			Fri			Fri	
	Sat			Sat			Sat	
	Sun			Sun			Sun	

Week	Day	Impact	Week	Day	Impact	Week	Day	Impact
10.	Mon		11.	Mon		12.	Mon	
	Tues			Tues			Tues	
	Wed			Wed			Wed	
	Thurs			Thurs			Thurs	
	Fri			Fri			Fri	
	Sat			Sat			Sat	
	Sun			Sun			Sun	

“It’s Good To Talk”: Therapy and You

There’s a moment tucked away towards the end of the second act of Die Hard where McClane is on the radio with Sgt Al Powell, the beat cop who’s inadvertently found himself first on scene at the clusterfuck McClane is caught up in at Nakatomi Plaza and ends up serving as his lifeline to the other cops and tacticians outside, as well as a form of support when the going gets tough by way of a two-way radio.

McClane is pulling shards of glass from his bare feet, beaten up but still trying to keep the banter going with Powell before the latter vulnerably puts forward his truth to the guy on the other side of the radio who he's never met before - that he took a desk job because he’d accidentally shot and killed a 13 year old child in the line of duty.

Critics to this day mark the scene up as an example of what sets Die Hard out differently to other action movies and other action heroes played by the likes of Sylvester Stallone, Arnold Schwarzenegger, or Chuck Norris from around that same time – Here were heroic character figures who looked like your or I and were both open and transparent with their feelings, who had flaws and talked about them.

There’s an even greater example within the movie in another conversation between McClane and Powell.

It’s the scene that absolutely drives home how Die Hard and inversely John McClane are different than your huge muscled, unkillable action heroes of the 1980s or the John Wayne types who were fearless and devoid of any other shade but stoic, machismo-drenched manliness.

It shows a hero who is scared, struggling, and is reaching out to another human being.

It's a scene that unifies McClane a little closer to you or me because he's vulnerable and he's out of his depth and he's really starting to feel that, and no action movies up to that point had taken the time in amongst the shooting and killing to stop and have a scene where the heroic protagonist talks about realising he should have been more supportive of his wife's personal and professional developments and accomplishments, and that he's beginning to face the reality that he's outnumbered / outgunned and unlikely to see her again. He asks Powell to tell her on his behalf that he is sorry.

Talking is good.

Talking is healthy and important when it comes to our mental health. Just look at the strength McClane was able to draw to carry on just by having a moment of vulnerability like that with Powell.

But we're going to go back to that word 'honest', again. It must be <u>authentic</u>. If it is not, it is meaningless and pointless. Ostensibly any sort of therapy is as good or as bad as the humans investing in on both sides – subject and support. The asset and the flaw are the same thing. How frustrating is that?

Even *more* frustrating is how to articulate it, I assure you.

Otto Preminger's still astonishing 1959 legal drama Anatomy of a Murder (an absolute 'peach' of a courtroom saga based on a real life 1952 murder case) remains famous for being one of the first legal dramas that reflected the inherit flaw 'jurisprudence' represents in the fundamental theories of law.

Jurisprudence is the core belief that the underpinnings of all law is destabilised by the very *fallibility* of human nature.

Each of us is intrinsically *individual* after all, right?

And that individuality brings varying sized dents, chips and scratches to the accepted notion of what is right and what is wrong.

It also puts a couple of hits on what is negotiable on a *moral* level between the two points (can theft be 'explained away' if you're stealing food to feed your starving child, for example?) and how we allow our own moral conjecture to sometimes *"get in the way"*.

That very 'human' component - the injection of one's own *subjective* position or emotive feeling - easily pollutes the rule of law because the elements of any case and how those elements are considered / interpreted is made up entirely by humans; the person prosecuting it, the person defending it, the witnesses, the jury, the judge and so forth. To really understand the jurisprudence that we're held to, we must accept the "*people*" of it all is the weak link within the legal foundations that binds us.

In many ways I feel that therapy in all its forms is intrinsically affected in the same way. It is built, it goes without saying, on human-to-human interaction and yet its success is weighted entirely by the very imperfect human element; how much one person invests in it truthfully and earnestly, how experienced the therapist or counsellor is, whether they're even truly listening to you versus covertly and quietly thinking about what they are going to have for dinner that night, the patient's accurate accounting of incidents and interactions, and so on and so forth.

Even now, writing this it feels like a truly bizarre 'nit-pick' to go with, doesn't it? I suppose you could argue that this is true of any profession – the goddamn 'human' element of it. I accept that. But in my experience, it is definitely a boon and a bust to therapy:

I've had counsellors and psychologists that have been excellent. I've had some that have been terrible. I've had mental health support where, looking back, it was highly evident that I was the problem with my malaise or distrust in engaging with the process openly or because I simply did not know how to communicate what it was I was feeling. I've also had counsellors and the like be so bad that I sometimes hope they've been struck off or found another occupation.

There was the psychotherapist who had recently graduated university and spent our time together showing me bikini-clad holiday photos of herself on her phone...

... whilst recommending the location of where she'd just come back from, or who filled out at least the first fifteen minutes of our forty minute sessions talking about her heavy drinking session the night before and trying to work out whether these were bars I'd previously frequented or not back when I was "well enough to go out" (her words).

On the flipside there was one counsellor who challenged my acceptance of my parents' regard of me in such a way that it was the first chink in the connecting chain that still inexplicably tied me to my family at that time despite all the abuse and emotional abandonment. I was speaking to her about my deep fear of marrying my now wife and having a family with her, infecting my children with mental ill health genetically and so on and so forth. Amid my 'ramble' I quoted my mother like she was a renowned expert in the field of parenting, explaining that "unconditional love" is not a "real thing". The counsellor asked for further clarification. I explained that when I was in my early teens I had got in trouble with the police whilst trying desperately to 'fit in' with the so-called cool kids at school. My mother told me that if I ever brought the police to her door again then I would be "disowned", and she would "put [me] into care". I said something about how she's meant to love me unconditionally, even when I've got in trouble or not done something right.

I still to this day, thirty-plus years on, remember her words because I took them as being an actual parenting standard for far too long. She said: "I don't have to love you unconditionally. That's not a real thing. Of course there's conditions. I'm not going to love you if you kill someone or if you embarrass this family. Why do I have to do that? Who says you must love someone if they clearly don't love you back by not doing what you need them to do?"

As a parent now myself I see the damage in any child believing that their parents' love comes with stipulations and small print.

Back then I had no point of comparison to know that this was far from a normal point of view and decidedly not a normal thing for an adult to say to their child. The counsellor on this occasion dug right in on that and kept putting it back to me that the comment spoke far more negatively of the person saying it than to the person it was being said to. I'll always remember this counsellor saying, "Have you ever put that remark back under a harder spotlight and looked at it again from a different angle – that it wasn't that you were deserving of such a remark but that the remark says more about the troubles the person saying it may possess emotionally?"

It feels so trite to simply say your therapy journey is only as effective as not just the work you put in but the therapist you get, but there's a lot of truth to that and the human fallibility of it all means that you can take the same incident / trauma / emotional conundrum to two different professionals and get two different perspectives and / or degrees of support in return.

In the mid-noughties I received a tearful phone-call from my grandma asking if she could have a chat. I rushed down to her home because a phone call of this ilk was so not like her at all. She explained that she had "done a stupid thing", going on to say that my father had come to her a few months back and discussed the idea of buying the council house she was living in and letting her live in it rent free thereafter but with a view to him having a "nest egg" to "sell on" when the time came where she was no longer around anymore. I asked what the problem was as I could only assume she'd be happy to take that deal.

My grandma explained that she initially agreed but she said it was on the sworn promise from my dad that he would not do any renovation work or changes to the property whilst she was living in it because she couldn't stand "mess", didn't like "change" and she was too old for "all the noise of workmen banging and clanging".

My dad assured her that she had nothing to worry about and she felt that she didn't...

... until she'd come to discover that very week it wasn't just my dad buying the house - it was an arrangement between my parents and my sister and her husband. They were going to buy it together, sell it and split the profits. My grandma started to cry and said she worried that she'd inadvertently taken part in something that would leave me "high and dry".

I said that none of that bothered me and she shouldn't worry about that but then she explained that my sister had been down to her home that day, telling her that once the paperwork was 'done' she would like my grandma to move out of her house "just for a month, maybe a month and a half" to the residential home for the elderly down the road "on respite" so that they could get some work done on the house. My grandma said that this wasn't what was agreed, and she knew if she moved out of the home she'd been in for *sixty years* (!) she wasn't going to get back in, and that they'd sell it out from underneath her. She hadn't signed anything yet, but she says she was being strong-armed into it and she couldn't face angering my father if she didn't.

Acting fast I utilised a solicitor ex-girlfriend at the time to help draw up a legal document my dad would have to sign explicitly agreeing to the original promise – no moving out, no renovation work, house can't be sold whilst my grandma's alive, etc. etc – and when my dad arrived to get my grandma to finalise the sale, he was shocked to his core to see me there and "involved" and even more so that there was now a counter-document in my grandma's hand she wanted him to sign first.

My dad blew an absolute gasket, as the saying goes. He started screaming at my grandma that she'd been "infected" by my "jealousy" due to my not being involved in "earning from the house" and that she clearly loved me more than him. I sat with my jaw open. I smoked at the time and excused myself to go for a cigarette outside. My dad followed me outside and slammed me up against the wall. "You smug little shit!" he shouted in my face. "I fucking hate you. I wish you'd never been born."

He drew his fist to hit me and as he threw it at my face, I caught it and clasped my hand around it tight.

My dad semi-froze at his action being interrupted mid-flow then he recalibrated, tipped his head back and spat directly into my face. "You're a fucking embarrassment to this family. I hate you." He then turned and stormed off to his car and sped out of the street as I dropped down onto my grandma's front step and tried to swipe the spit from my eye and nose with my sleeve.

I told a counsellor this for the first time as a way of trying to articulate that as horrible a moment as that was in some ways it helped amidst the hurt because it validated what I felt my family thought about me. This counsellor simply replied "Why did you get involved though? What made you think you had a right to get in the middle of that arrangement between your father and his mother? Are you able to see where your father's anger came from?"

Flash forwards a decade and change, later that same incident got dropped in a therapy session as an almost aside and a completely different counsellor took the anecdote and put forward the notion that it was more revealing of my father's character, insecurities, absence of integrity and the like. "If we were looking at proportionate reactions to upsetting actions on the adversity scale that we've been looking at together, do you think your dad would have scored well there? No. So why should you hold yourself accountable to his failings in that instance?"

The same incident, the same guilt, the same upset, all carried across two different points in time and two different emotional lines of thought and support drawn from it, depending on the professional being spoken to. That's the mental health 'jurisprudence' I'm trying to dig into here.

There is so much at play in getting talking therapies of all kinds to land right and fit correctly with you.

That includes measuring your expectations accordingly.

But also understanding the different types of therapy and the different roles a psychiatrist plays to a psychologist and a therapist and or counsellor to them both.

One of the most recurrent complaints I heard from people time and again when speaking about their mental health support is how "ineffective" they found counselling to be because the counsellor frequently didn't "have the answers" or "give proper guidance", without necessarily realising that in most cases it isn't the counsellors' job to give you the solutions or steps to take on the journey. It is to non-intrusively help you find your way there yourself. In most cases a CBT counsellor will be well-trained and experienced in specifically *not* giving opinions or being seen to directly guide you, but to make you feel like you guided yourself there instead. Being prepared and knowledgeable about this from the outset will set your expectation correctly.

All of this is before you even consider the very real mental health support *crisis* that we're facing right now.

And make no bones about it, it *is* a crisis.

The country is in an economic decline that is facilitating an enormous and devastating cost of living crisis made worse after surviving a global pandemic the likes of which we've not seen internationally in my lifetime, for sure. This alone is having a detrimental effect on people's mental health, but then you add to this the sharp increases in workplace related stress and the fact emotional impacts specific to that are now wider in the age demographics affected than ever before [for example; a survey by Cigna International Health in 2023 of around 12,000 workers internationally showed that 91% of employees aged just 18 to 24 years old are suffering from work-specific stress and burn-out symptoms] and the fact suicide amongst men is higher than it has ever been.

There are not enough trained professionals and therefore there are not enough available appointments with accessible support services. Most definitely here in the UK.

The Care Quality Commission (CQC) believe there were serious mental health incidents (self-harm, suicide attempts, psychosis, etc.) occurring two times every hour throughout 2023, not counting the ever-flowing need for 'impactive but functional' community mental health support requirements (depression, stress, anxiety, etc.) and there simply isn't the staff available to combat or assist.

As it stands currently at the time of writing this, within my own community, there are waiting times of three months *minimum* to access mental health support provisions (i.e. talking therapies) through your GP on the NHS. The immediate focus is on having your 'triaged' by a trained professional before then so that the most accurate signposting for support occurs.

Even *when* it arrives it can feel a little underwhelming and almost immediately ineffective. I have had experiences of counselling, experiences shared by people I spoke to for this book, where the course of counselling is so short (for example, the average person experiencing quite debilitating employment-related stress to a level that they have been signed off from work can routinely expect to receive six thirty-to-forty minute sessions weekly or fortnightly – with *no* guarantee of extension of treatment) it feels almost pointless in being able to effectively tackle the core issues.

Let me break that down with some illustrations for better effect.

Yeah, I fiddled around on my phone's photo app with my finger. Cut me some slack, okay? I'm an analogue man in a digital world, alright?

Using myself as a short case study:

I was brought up in an abusive home environment which caused extreme detrimental harm to my esteem and how I was able to formulate and maintain friendships and relationships, as well as how I saw the world and my place in it which in turn affected the work environments that I went into and how I succeeded in them.

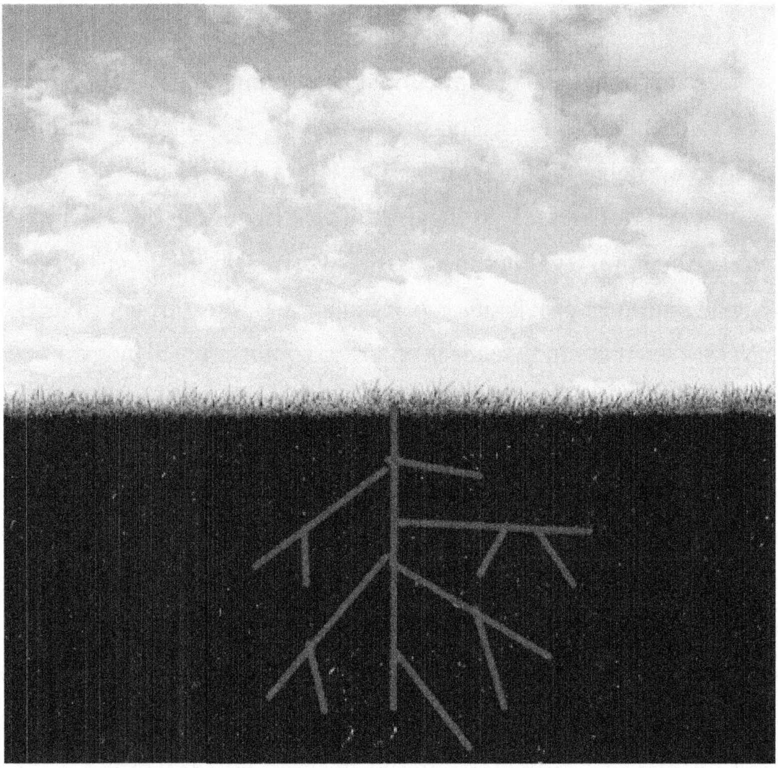

All these things stirred around in a cup together would give me bouts of depression so severe I did not want to live, or I would 'ghost' myself through my life. The therapeutic ideal would be to simply reach down, grab at the roots (my past abuse and my self-esteem) and tend to them.

However, all too frequently, by the time we're accessing therapy whether that's through personal choice or availability the roots have grown weeds, and the weeds are a little out of control and impactive on getting to the roots themselves.

We're talking insomnia, alcohol or drug misuse, relationship problems, etc.

All of which are driving to increase or inflame the mental ill health issue(s). Hence why we're seeking support.

We need a little help in getting the proverbial garden back under control so we can get to the 'roots'.

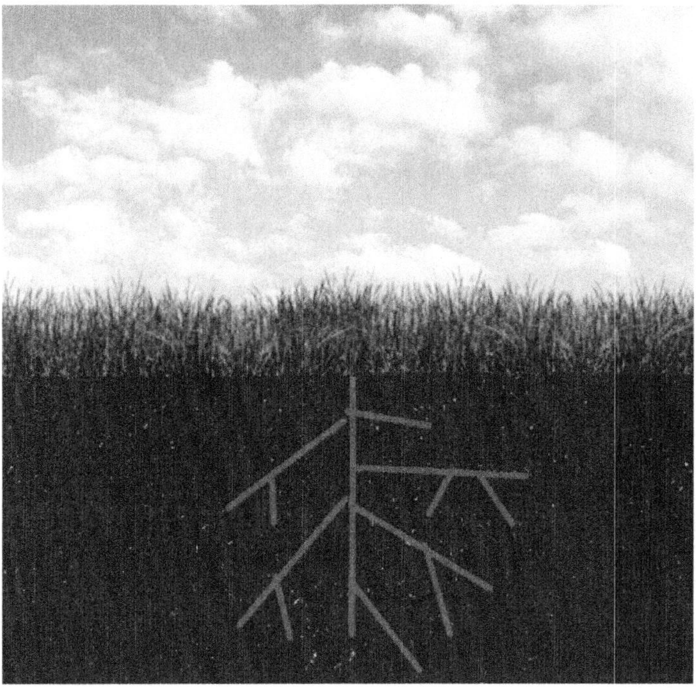

You leave any area overgrown and uncared for and it is just going to inadvertently become a 'dumping ground' for other people's waste, dog muck and so on and so forth.

Before you know it, your insomnia and your alcohol consumption are impacting your work.

Or as is the common cry more and more nowadays, work is exploiting you to the point that you're overworked, under-supported, stressed and heading for burn-out.

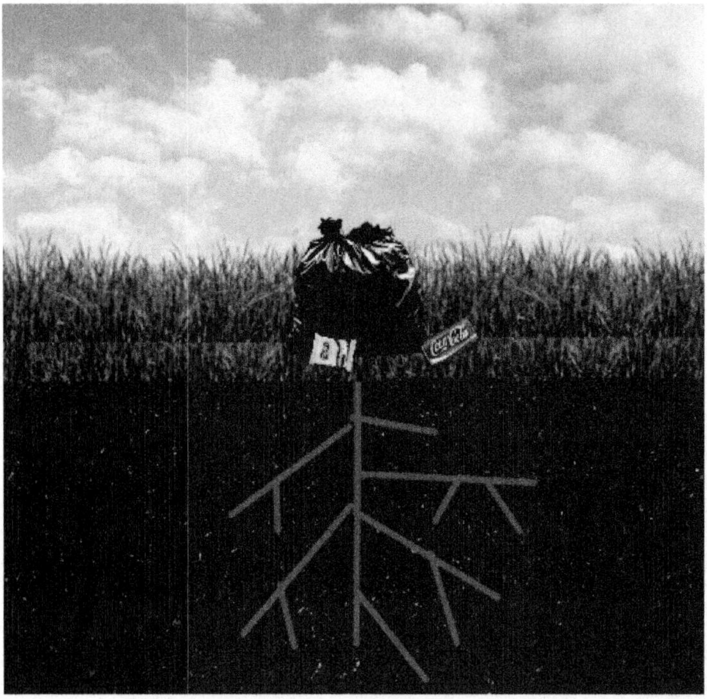

It's 'rubbish' you can do without.

Rubbish stacked on top of already pre-existing problems and your therapy sessions (small in number as they are anyway) start to feel like an adhesive bandage over a gunshot wound.

You're just dealing with the impacts of the week and how they've affected with you without ever really getting down to the core of the problem.

All too quickly we'll either come to the end of therapy or disengage from it without really feeling we've gotten anywhere and that's because by the time we've picked up the "rubbish" and "cut back the grass", it's time to stop.

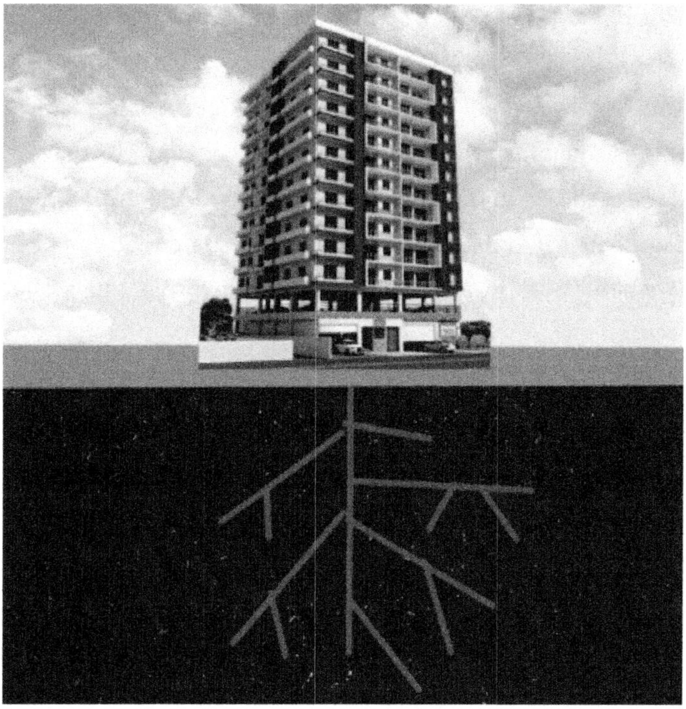

Frequently we will just 'muster on' and bury the roots – concrete 'em down and move on.

We tried to get the roots 'out' and dealt with and it didn't work so... yeah, fuck it huh? It was worth a shot.

Instead, we just build on top and try to forget about it.

Before you know it you can forget Joni Mitchell's "paradise" because it's your mental health issues that have been "paved" and structures built atop of them – friendships, work, family, children, financial obligations, health, etc.

But these can't exactly be the strongest of foundations to have built upon, can they?

And there lies the risk that the structures could start to weaken and even bring the goddamn building down...

If I'd been 'cleverer' for the purposes of synergy the building in the last example would have been the building from Die Hard, wouldn't it?

But I'm not that skilled so let's just move on...

So, it goes without saying that by the time you land in front of a trained professional for your handful of allocated support, you've got to be prepared to hit the ground running and 'do the work'.

What does that look like and how can you do that though – especially when, to put it in the bluntest possible terms, you can't be *fucked* and just working your way up to asking for help was a task and a half in the first place?

Firstly, you've got to take a second with yourself and your thoughts and you've got to do some 'gardening' on your own, trying to separate out some of the impactors (money issues, work related strain) and align yourself with correct avenues of support for those matters (speaking to the support departments at your bank, Citizens Advice Bureau or employment-specific organisations like ACAS) so that the 'grass' is thinned out enough for the 'roots' to be accessed from the get-go.

Or to put it in our reoccurring Die Hard parlance, you've got to kill your way through the thankless 'henchmen' to get to the real 'meat' behind it all, namely Alan Rickman's legendary villain Hans Gruber and his second-in-command Karl (Alexander Godunov – a real life Russian ballet dancer who defected to the US and became an actor!).

You remember all those thankless henchmen, don't you?

Sure you do.

There's stress / depression / anxiety impactor representatives like Gruber's lower-tier team-members:

Bruno Doyon's Franco, Andreas Wisniewski's Tony, Joey Plewa as Alexander, Lorenzo Caccialanza as Marco, Gerard Bonn's Kristoff, Gary Roberts as Heinrich, Hans Buhringer's Fritz, Dennis Hayden as Eddie, the celebrated stuntman turned cult bit-player Al Leong as Uli, and the demon from the painting in Ghostbusters II (Wilhelm von Homburg) as James.

Don't fret immediately if you don't even feel well enough to separate out some of those impactors and align yourself with correct avenues of support elsewhere for them.

That can be something you discuss early on with your counsellor, and they can help signpost you to separate the impactors away from the underlying issues.

After all, it favours them to be able to get to the primary stuff. That way together you can then set small, achievable goals to work on each session as opposed to the time spent with you just venting out everything that's impacted you or affected you between your appointment(s), which has frequently been the barrier in therapy for me – the sessions don't feel sufficient in length nor number to fight back against the wave of knock-downs and struggles I was facing week-to-week, day-to-day resultant from the originating issue that got me assigned to therapy in the first place.

To enter therapy and draw from it effectively you need to be in the 'correct' position to be able to do so. To assess your position, you've got to ask yourself the *hard* questions. Don't worry, you don't even need to think them up. I've put them down here for you and all you must do is write them out on a bit of paper and scribble instinctively your reactive thoughts to each one:

1. *Can I open myself up to talk about the things that are difficult and personal that are affecting me?*
2. *If not, why not? Is there anything that I can immediately identify as being a barrier to doing this?*
3. *Am I ready at this point with where I am mentally and emotionally to explore and, in some cases, challenge the things that are difficult and personal which are affecting me and my behaviour(s)?*
4. *What do I want to get out of therapy?*
5. *What scares me about taking part in therapy?*

Your answers can help you in self-assessing whether you are in the right place to engage with therapy but if you do, the instinctive answers you've written out can greatly help you very early on with a good therapist / counsellor to lay down strong foundations and set useful goals.

Therapy sessions are your time to talk about what is impacting you and you should never allow yourself to be told what you can or cannot talk about. You should however have a willingness to be guided – especially back round to things you've tried to skirt past or not address which a trained professional is identifying as a causation factor on your ill health or struggles.

Going back to the 'human factor' and the 'good and bad of it' all when it comes to therapy, if you put the work in you must remember you have a controlling stake in its value; if the type of therapy and counselling isn't working for you tell your therapist, if the therapist themselves isn't someone you feel you're gelling with or feel that you can trust then ask to be assigned to an alternative.

Sure, amid the crisis we're facing now, you'll face a delay whilst this is recalibrated, but it is ultimately about getting the best and most effective support available to you.

There's no point coming away after eight weeks still feeling the same way or worse but at least being able to recognise your psychotherapist looks very good in a bikini with a cocktail in her hand.

The "3 T's" Strategy

A mountain only looks insurmountable from the bottom. It certainly looks more achievable when you're halfway up and it feels suddenly very feasible to surmount when you're a hundred or so metres from the peak, right?

We use 'mountains' as visual or verbal metaphors a lot for tasks and problems, don't we? Mountains of debt. Mountains of work. Mountains of knockbacks. It's interesting that we do that because a mountain doesn't move. *We* do. We reach for it time and again to exemplify the weight and size of our difficulty, reflective of it as this great big barrier that's stopping us or intimidating us in our paths, yet routinely we simply move up, over or around it.

The size is the thing.

I was in a job that I enjoyed and felt very comfortable in. It was a public, uniformed organisation that offered me an opportunity to really let loose with the twenty plus years of accrued skills in my specialist field, to train and mentor others in said field which I was passionate about and, most importantly, to advance in areas that I had great interest in.

[If you're thinking that said "uniformed organisation" sure does sound like something that rhymes with 'faa-lease nervous' but can't possibly be identified as such on legal grounds then... the prize is in the post to you!]

Then I made the mistake of reporting wrongdoing. A much younger and more popular colleague committed acts that were illegal and inherently dishonest. I was put in a position where I had to speak honestly about what had occurred – and overnight the ramifications of doing so were overwhelmingly negative and incredibly impactive.

I was ostracised by most of my colleagues. I was isolated and abandoned for future progression. I was targeted by upper management. And worst of all when I spoke out about all this the 'targeting' only got worse. I would get double (sometimes triple) the workload of any other member of staff, I would work twelve hour shifts often without speaking a single word to another person and I would see my professional achievements taken from me and given to somebody else to take credit for. It was explained to me again and again that I was being "worked to quit". The organisation didn't want me because they saw me as a "grass", but they had no grounds to fire me, so they were going to keep up this treatment until I resigned. They'd done it many times before. They didn't see why they couldn't do it again.

I refused to resign and became resolute in rolling into work every day and doing my job, often in extremely lonely and sometimes unsafe conditions. I just refused to give them what they wanted. The cost however was that I became deeply miserable, and my depression returned aggressively, affecting my sleep and my mood.

I had very young children by this point, and I felt that I had to 'keep going' for them at the very least. Then I found out that I had been passed over for progression again but this time in a very nakedly corrupt manner, and that the opportunity I went for had been handed to the very person I originally spoke out about – someone who had carried out sex acts on work premises, openly cheated on exams and bragged about it, had an affair with the investigator looking into her misconduct... I could go on and on. I'm not even touching the sides. I asked myself the question of what it said about *me* that someone like that could be continually rewarded and given opportunities to flourish in a uniformed public service (one the public no longer held confidence in, justifiably so given what I witnessed) whilst I was punished, bullied, and purposefully mistreated for speaking out about wrongdoing in an organisation that continually claims to value people doing just that.

I didn't like the answer.

Before I knew it the bottom was dropping out of my world again, mentally. And the 'domino effect' we're all familiar with kicked in – I was so stressed that it was affecting my sleep, my sleep was affecting my energy levels and my mood, my thought processes were overwhelming negative and without value, I stopped eating properly, I was unable to get into work because I fluctuated between being too utterly exhausted to move and too angry at the injustices I was faced with to want to leave the house, fearful that I would go into work and start punching the people that had belittled me or went out of their way to handicap my advancement.

The ill health affected my drive, my relationships and the like. Then the concerns of being able to pay bills if I stayed off sick too much longer raised their head. Our savings were getting depleted. Whether I could feed my sons the following month started to weigh down upon me. The pressure increased and increased and with it the feeling that I was having heart attacks – I would frequently have to get down on all fours and gasp for air to avoid passing out and banging my head on something.

My wife would try to talk to me, and I would go off on enormous conspiratorial rants, the type of which even I would catch myself listening to from the inside out and think "Okay, calm down Oliver Stone! Jesus!" Mid listing of the latest additions and developments that were piling up on top of all the stuff that had made me sick my wife simply put her hand on my chest and very quietly said "Stop."

I stopped speaking.

"We're going to deal with this. Then we're going to deal with that." she said. "Okay? We can't deal with everything at once. So, we're going to deal with the first thing, then the next thing. And we don't deal with the next thing until we've dealt with the first thing. Deal?"

And in that moment ~~her~~ my 'Three T' method was born:

This. Then that.

This. **T**hen **t**hat.

By that point in my mental health ride, I'd already reached a juncture where I had started to believe that mental health difficulties were never cured, they were simply outpaced and controlled. I just didn't have a strong enough understanding as to *how* to do that. Suddenly I did – by applying a 'this, then that' approach.

If you think about it, you wouldn't wake up one day without ever having ran more than five miles and simply decide to go out and run a marathon. And not only that but run it at full sprint. That's impossible. You don't have the stamina and there's no way that pace could ever be maintained. So, with that same principle, you can't simply wake up one morning and look at your depression / anxiety / stress / exhaustion etc. and simply go "Get fucked!" then run off at high speed. You'll run out of steam and the ol' black cloud (or whatever your representing visual aid is) will slowly, methodically crawl up at its usual pace and engulf you.

It's about the small regular steps.

There's a reason why Aesop's Fable of 'The Tortoise & The Hare' still hangs around and resonates as something of value all these years on. And when I say "all these years" it's important to remember he first cranked out this story sometime between 620 and 564 BCE. (I should know what it's like to have that degree of impact as a storyteller carry with time because a good many years ago, I was in my local pub, talking about a date that went wrong and I used the expression "Now I know I'm more Cess Pitt than Brad Pitt..." and loads of people burst out laughing. The next week when I went into the pub the landlord said "Hey, it's Cess Pitt!" and gave me my pint of lager for free. So... yeah... you could say I recognise Aesop's skill and influence.)

The problem with 'The Tortoise & The Hare' I tend to find is that 'some' people draw the wrong moral from the parable because it gets commonly associated with the atypical folklore interpretations attached to these sorts of tales; that trickery and ingenuity are best employed to better or overcome a stronger opponent.

One of my best friends told me recently that even they thought the moral of said fable was that the tortoise "mind-fucked" the hare into thinking he was "slower and not as good as he actually was". I continue to be his friend presently, but I'm not going to lie – I'm kind of struggling to move past this.

The moral is screamingly evident (sorry mate!), namely that you can be considerably more successful by taking your time and doing things slowly and consistently rather than acting carelessly, recklessly, or too quickly to have given full regard to your circumstances.

The *this* and the *that* is intrinsically individual to <u>you</u>: If you're at a point where your mental ill health has overwhelmed you to the extent that you can't get out of bed, that you've literally blinked away an entire day – the *this* is to simply work on getting out of bed. That's it. The showering, the brushing your teeth, getting dressed and what not? That's a whole lot of *that*. Each of those gets broken down to become a *this* individual of each other later down the line.

Small steps, you see?

Don't rout yourself with what's going on outside of your house until you have taken control of looking after yourself inside of it. The pressures of your employer trying to get you back to work, your friends demanding that you 'shake it off' and 'get back out in the world', the managing of your finances... they don't go away, but they become easier when you're sleeping better, eating well, and closing off the funnel flow of stresses to a manageable stream that you're in control of.

We're not going to enter a state of denial as if these problems and impactors aren't there and don't need dealt with. What we're going to do is exert a degree of control over them that will serve as beneficial to us. Each degree of control is a 'step'. Each 'step' is distance between you and your 'cloud' (or 'dog', 'tank', however you manifest it). That's why we list them, rate them based on how much they're impacting our ability to function, prioritise them correctly and then we work through them.

One. Then the other.

Multitasking is for *fools* in this instance. As the age old saying goes; it's better to do one thing very well than many things just adequately or poorly. You don't need another cheeky Die Hard analogy here, do you? You don't – but you want one anyway, don't you?

Okay. By now you know *fine well* John McClane's success lay in stealthily moving around the skyscraper, picking off one bad guy at a time where possible and not just bombing into a room and trying to kill all of them at once.

That's how we are with the impactors upon on our mental health.

We go after them one at a time, floor by floor through the Nakatomi Plaza of our brain.

How we work our list requires us to really just put a pen to a piece of paper and get it all 'out' in the first instance – all of the shit that's sitting on top of us and making it hard for us to breathe; the work stress, the relationship troubles, the money difficulties, the feelings of hopelessness that leave you lying in bed for days on end not eating or washing.

Really don't hold back on yourself if you can help it.

It should look a little something like this, perhaps:

I'm so burnt out with work I'm exhausted.

I spend all day in bed.

Friends have started to give up on me because I keep cancelling on them.

I'm off sick from work.

Work are not being supportive.

I often think that I'd be better off dead.

I'm exhausted but I can't sleep.

I can't stop thinking and overthinking.

I worry work are going to sack me.

I don't know how I am going to pay my bills etc. if I lose my job.

Now we rate our list based on the impact it is having on our life and our ability to function on a day-to-day level. Let's say **5** is incredibly impactive and **1** is that it's not particular impactive, but it is sitting there in the background as a low-level anxiety-agitator.

I'm so burnt out with work I'm exhausted.	4
I spend all day in bed.	5
Friends have started to give up on me because I keep cancelling	4
on them.	4
I'm off sick from work.	3
Work are not being supportive.	5
I often think that I'd be better off dead.	5
I'm exhausted but I can't sleep.	4
I can't stop thinking and overthinking.	3
I worry work are going to sack me.	3
I don't know how I am going to pay my bills etc. if I lose my job.	3

Now what we're going to do is give immediate focus to the issues listed that are causing the highest impact and we're going to see if we can prioritise them correctly so the tackling of one will affect the impact scale or diminish entirely one of the others.

I spend all day in bed.	5
I often think that I'd be better off dead.	5
I'm exhausted but I can't sleep.	5

The picture is looking ever so slightly clearer now, isn't it?

Just on the smallest of scales.

Now, obviously the feeling that you'd be better off dead is huge and hugely unhelpful. It's incredibly impactive and likely playing a large part in the other two elements. But we're unlikely to get help or move slightly away from the feeling from our bed and we need to *start small* anyway, so we look at our immediate shortlist and we could perhaps rank our priorities in this order:

I spend all day in bed.	5	1
I often think that I'd be better off dead.	5	3
I'm exhausted but I can't sleep.	5	2

Controversial ranking perhaps? Yet here's the thing; that feeling of negativity and suicidal ideation is being polluted by how our emotions and our brain are operating on such little sleep. We are getting little sleep to the point of it being so impactive because we are not tired. We're not tired because we are spending all day in bed, not doing anything to tire ourselves out.

The stark truth of it at this stage is that even the smallest of moves outside of your bed is going to feel enormously exhaustive *anyway* so we set our 'this' as simply getting out of bed. Not to go anywhere. Not to do anything in particular or see anyone. Just get out of bed and look at a different wall.

The 'this' is merely getting out of bed.

Do you see how it works?

Once out of bed, you've accomplished the 'this' and now you're going to pick a new one from your 'that' list. Something that is a slight push above what you've not been managing to do up to this point but will serve well to tire you out – cook a meal, take a shower, do some light housework like hoovering or ironing.

You get tired, you'll sleep even if it's snatched. An hour here or there. Twenty minutes. It's more restorative even at that tiny amount than the amount you were getting before which was close to zero.

By getting out of bed we've tired ourselves even just a little so that we are now napping at worst or stealing *some* restorative sleep back at best. Inadvertently, we may well have ticked off a 'that' without even realising or before it even became a 'this:

~~I spend all day in bed.~~

I often think that I'd be better off dead.

~~I'm exhausted but I can't sleep.~~

You're up out of bed. You've made a move towards getting washed and maybe even putting some clothes on. You can now put your focus on picking up the phone and reaching out to explore why you feel you would be better off dead, by speaking to a doctor or support services like The Samaritans. Doing that is a massive step and you may feel you have to coax yourself into doing so. Don't undersell the weight of feeling attached to reaching out.

If that is the only 'this' you accomplish that day that is more than enough and you should feel really, really fucking *proud* of yourself.

Once you've done that, let yourself have a moment. Reward yourself in some way. Try and avoid alcohol or drugs. We've discussed why. You *know* why. Don't make me be the goddamn parent here. Maybe treat yourself to something like a new item of clothing or a film. Order yourself a nice meal. You know? Stop with the usual McDonalds order and spritz yourself a Burger King for a change. You're *worth it* – You deserve it. I jest. Junk food ain't great. You get the picture though.

Just make sure you really take that time to acknowledge to yourself that whilst treading water in a dark, deep ocean of very weighty feelings and pressures without any feeling of control, you reached out and took a modicum of *charge*. And that is worth a lot. Then once you've done that...

Head back to the list, look at what was next on the priority line...

I'm so burnt out with work I'm exhausted.	4
Friends have started to give up on me because I keep cancelling	4
on them.	4
I'm off sick from work.	4
I can't stop thinking and overthinking.	

... and **start again**.

I use the principle of 'this then that' as the underpinning of everything when staying in control of my mental health in all its peaks and troughs. It has become so integral to how I go about tasks or challenges specific to bouts of depression, low mood, or anxiety. You know those adverts you used to see of celebrities endorsing stuff and there was always a run where someone would go "Hell, I have so much faith in [such and such] that I bought shares in the company myself!"

Well… I believe so significantly in 'this then that' as being at the core of what I must do to best manage my own mental well-being that I got it tattooed on myself!

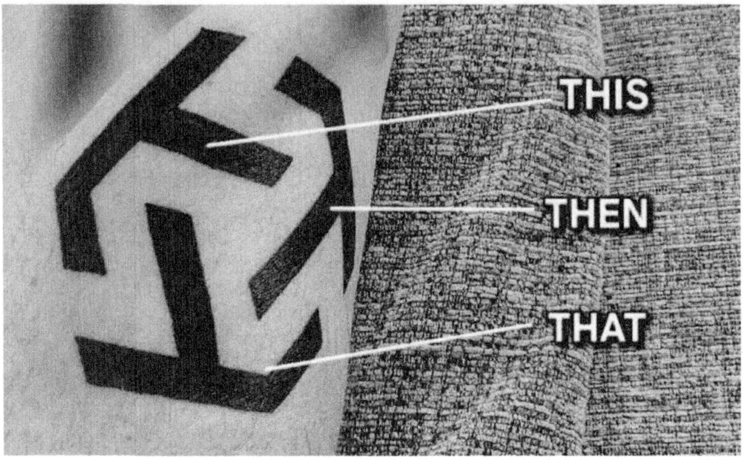

Challenging The Catastrophe

I once spent just shy of three weeks on my sofa. Quite literally. I stayed there all day. I slept there at night. The only movement I would make would be to the kitchen to get myself a drink and put a cheese slice between two pieces of bread. I drank and smoked heavily whilst watching old kung fu films and late 1970s but mostly 1980s creature features (shout out to Lewis Teague's Alligator and Larry Cohen's Q: The Winged Serpent!). What few friends I had would try to check in, but they'd mostly get ignored. My [now widowed by this point] grandma would take a bus and a metro just to get to my flat, bringing me food and trying to get me to cross the road and go for lunch or go for a walk with her. I'd make excuses not to, cry after she left with the guilt I felt at her coming all that way just to see me wallowing like this then reject her help... and after she was gone I'd drink the guilt away.

I washed in the kitchen sink every morning because I didn't want to go into the bathroom where the mirror was as I could not bear looking at my reflection or catching sight of myself. One friend recognised what the 'set-up' here appeared to be and would come round every five or six days with a bag of food and cigarettes, push to sit and watch a film with me and then leave without applying any pressure for me to speak about 'things' or anything.

My weight was plummeting, and I started to fixate on the idea that I could just waste away on the sofa.

Waste away in front of a triple-bill of the 1987 'Ozploitation' killer crocodile movie Dark Age, Chuck Russell's remake of The Blob and John Frankenheimer's Prophecy which is meant to be an environmental disaster horror film by the way but let's not kid ourselves here people:

It's a movie about a giant mutant killer bear and has a scene in it where the bear smashes somebody inside of a sleeping bag off a tree and they explode into bloodied feathers!

(Fun fact whilst we're talking about irresponsible alcohol consumption– Did you know that *allegedly* John Frankenheimer quit drinking once and for all after decades as a functioning alcoholic because he started getting royalty cheques for a 1979 giant mutant killer bear movie he had no clear memory of having directed?)

I'd ended up in this position because another toxic relationship had ended badly and within the same week, I'd been made redundant from a job I'd been in less than a year. My parents and my sister were being worse than usual towards me, culminating in my father handing my brother-in-law twenty pounds in front of me and telling him fair was fair. I asked what this was about, and I learnt that my family had placed bets on me losing the job within one year of getting it. An argument arose about what I felt was them treating me like a joke and my sister replied "You *are* though. I mean look at your life."

This was two weeks before Christmas and it led to me spending Christmas alone in my flat not speaking to my family, eating nothing but a Chocolate Orange my Grandma had bought me, whilst drinking heavily and chain-smoking my way through the Indiana Jones trilogy.

(The fourth movie that fucked the perfect run was five months or so away from landing.)

I fell into a depression that I struggled to pull out of, and I was still years out from formulating a better understanding of my mental health.

Christmas Day alone turned into those three weeks on the sofa, just about existing. And then it culminated in me attempting to attempt suicide.

On the day in question, I indulged in my usual mental and emotional self-flagellation whilst sat watching C.H.U.D.

(It stands for 'Cannibalistic Humanoid Underground Dwellers' just in case you weren't aware).

Man, could you have imagined if C.H.U.D had been the *last* movie I'd ever seen?

Now, I love C.H.U.D don't get me wrong. Big fan in fact.

Of all the movies that features a load of great actors who'd go on to do big things taking a movie about people in rubber suits pretending to be mutant cannibals *way* too seriously, it is probably my favourite.

But I don't know that looking back I'd have wanted it to be the *last* movie I ever saw.

During these three weeks a mate had asked if he could give my phone number to one of his girlfriend's friends as she had seen my photo on his Facebook page and inexplicably liked the look of me – this was back in an era when your Facebook news feed used to be your friend's actual day-to-day content and not sponsored adverts about grout cleaner or non-stop clips of that barely amusing Liverpudlian fella doing "spontaneous" interactions with people at his stand-up comedy shows. Yes, I *am* that old. Yes, I *am* aware your sponsored ads are frequently based on your search engine algorithms on the internet. And yes, I *am* continually in search of a suitably impressive grout cleaner that can act up to my robust expectations.

I kind of demurred but said friend went and did it anyway and in the thick of my depression and heavy drinking I would text with this girl, and daydream away about her as if she was this 'beacon' that was going to lead me out of my fug. She was something I could 'use' as a reason to get my shit together and go on dates and all that blather. (Not good foundations for starting any relationship, for what it's worth!)

We'd text almost daily.

We got along well.

She thought I was funny.

I was faking a whole heap of normality and doing so well enough that we arranged to go on a date.

This was suddenly my reason to get off my arse and kick myself into gear because this girl was beautiful, and she seemed to like me and...

... three days away from meeting up for a drink down the coast together she cancelled on me.

I tried to rearrange but she blew me off. Within a day of cancelling, she did what the 'kidz' these days refer to as "ghosting". My friend soon explained to me that it turned out this girl's family knew my sister and when she made passing reference to knowing me and that she was going to go for drinks with me, my sister told this girl to "steer clear".

In fact, what she actually told her was that I'd "been in the military for all of five minutes and it had fucked [my] head up", that it had "left me unable to hold down a job" and that I had "no friends and spent all [my] time wallowing and watching films."

Obviously, the fact that I found this out whilst wallowing and watching films did not help my cause. I'll admit that. So, of course this girl ran a mile. And I was left feeling humiliated and hurt. When your own family is actively working against you what chance do you have? And it was that *one* single thought that set me off.

From that one thought I was able to take it and catastrophise it to a very nearly fatal extent. Let me show you how. See if you see anything of yourself and how you process thoughts and feelings in your own lowest mood. The core details can be switched out to your own, but ultimately in much the same way that a building is going to come down if it is built on poor foundations (Remember that? Chapter 6! *C'mon*. Keep up!) there can be a whole heap of trouble from putting an unchecked negative thought on top of an unchallenged negative feeling again and again and again, until the 'teeter' turns to a 'topple':

My own family is actively working against me having any chance at happiness. What chance do I have at happiness when my family are championing me to fail? What is it about me that makes my own family hate me? What did I do and what do I continue to do that invites such mockery and criticism from them? Your family is meant to know you best and if they see me this way, no wonder everyone else sees me this way too. I'm just a joke to people. Everyone pushes me around and exploits me. That's why I keep struggling in work – because there's a total disconnect between how I want to be treated by people and how people think I deserve to be treated. I'm not deserved of respect. I want to be great enough at something that it almost demands respect from people, especially my family. Why can't I accept that there's great people in life and there's also-rans and I'm an also-ran? No one cares about me. How on earth am I going to find the drive to find another job when I am inevitably just going to fuck it up and piss people off in it? If I don't find another job I'm not going to be able to keep my home. Where am I going to live? How am I going to attract a girlfriend if I don't have a job or somewhere to live? I'm not getting any younger, thinner or more attractive so why would anyone want to go out with me with all the mental health baggage I carry? Who's going to want to marry me or have children with me? I'm just an also-ran who wishes for greatness, hated by his own family and without any friends, who's just existing rather than living and it hurts so bad each day to wake up and be reminded of this. If I wasn't around anymore my parents wouldn't have to keep dealing with me as an 'embarrassment'. My sister would be happy as she can go back to being the sole focus of my parents' attention. I would finally be at peace from having to face what a loser I am. I don't have a wife or children so it isn't like there's anyone that's going to miss me anyway...

... and before you knew it, I'd eyed the garden hose in the back yard outside my window and recalled reading somewhere that death from carbon monoxide poisoning through your car exhaust fumes was a pretty easy and painless way to go.

That is some bullshit right there, by the way.

As a rule, we all accept that getting advice – especially of a medical, emotional, mental health nature - off internet search engines is generally a ***terrible*** thing, don't we?

In the same way I often think back to a criminal who was once before a US court for sending an ineffective letter bomb to his ex-employer because they "made [him] feel like a failure" only to have the judge say to him "Well, it didn't go off so they may have had a point about you!", I think we need to really shine the 'bullshit' spotlight on those giving 'advice' or 'guidance' around best suicide methods because those fuckers are still around, tip-tapping nonsense out onto the internet... exploiting vulnerable people in a state of emotional catastrophe, like me that day.

I didn't have a garage or an enclosed space, so I knew that I would need to be somewhere where the engine could run undisturbed for enough time to fill up my car with carbon monoxide. I took the hose and drove down to Tynemouth Priory late that night, with a spot in mind of an old semi-abandoned overflow car park that was tucked almost out of sight and where I could sit feasibly undiscovered until at least daylight.

I pulled into the area to find another car parked up in the far left corner. I parked up away from them and needed to wait for them to leave before I could get out and get set up.

They flashed their lights at me.

This startled me but I chose to ignore them.

I hunkered down in my driver's seat and hoped they would leave soon. They didn't. But another car pulled in and parked directly opposite them.

This new car switched off its engine then flashed its lights twice and...

Look, you know where this is going so let's just *get there*, okay? Yes, right in front of my eyes the driver of the first car got out and his female passenger come round and started to perform oral sex on him whilst he stood in front of his beaming headlights.

I looked over to the car that had last arrived and could see that the driver was doing something with his out-of-sight hand to himself that indicated masturbation.

I hastily switched my engine on and exited out of there and pulled up to the main car park overlooking the sea. It was empty and I alighted and went and sat on a bench close to the edge of the cliff.

I remember thinking to myself that I wished I had the courage to just jump. I smoked a couple of cigarettes and heard someone approaching so I went to return to my car, just as an older man wrapped up against the cold came walking along the thin pathway towards me with his dog.

He said hello and I responded as I climbed inside my car and shut the door quickly. He had to pass tight to my car and in doing so he would have seen the hose on the passenger seat along with a roll of thick tape to eventually hold it in position.

I recollect seeing his pace slow and almost stutter to a stop as he passed the passenger side window. I could see him stop at the back of my car and he stood there for the longest time before turning and coming round to my window. He tapped on it, and I opened the car door slightly.

"Are you okay?" he asked.

I nodded.

"Could I borrow a cigarette?" he said.

I reached over, picked up the pack and handed them to him. He lit a cigarette, handed the pack to me, and stood holding the door frame open. After what I had just witnessed further down the hill, I was convinced he was about to come on to me sexually or proposition me to do something to him.

He exhaled his smoke and smiled, looking past me at the hose and tape on the passenger seat.

"You sure you're okay, son? You're not up to anything daft, are you?"

I tried to speak but this agonising lump developed in my throat and when I swallowed heavy, warm tears fell down my cheeks.

The man nodded, turned, and pulled his dog closer on the lead so it was now next to my car door. "Give him a stroke. You'll feel better. Trust me."

I faked a smile and reached down (after making eye contact long enough with him to definitely make sure he was referring to the dog – because after what I'd just seen minutes earlier, you can't be too careful can you?), stroking his Labrador down its head and onto its neck.

[Seriously, pack it in at the back – This is meant to be a big emotional moment here, and you's are ruining it with your sniggering and your innunendo-isms! Come on. Let's get back to the 'drama'. 3... 2... 1... And we're back!]

"What's his name?" I asked.

"Oliver." The man replied.

I kept stroking the dog and Oliver seemed to like what I was doing.

Eventually the man knelt to meet my eye line and suggested I go home. "Why not go home, get some sleep, and see how you feel in the morning? And if you don't feel any better, I'm back out with Oliver along here at half eight. You can come walk with us if you like?"

I was too embarrassed to do anything other than nod and turn the ignition on the engine to start the car up. I couldn't even commit suicide properly, I thought to myself. I ended up accidentally going 'dogging' and then getting interrupted by a twilight dog walker and... I drove home, flopped down on the sofa, and decided to kill myself tomorrow instead. I never saw that man again. Or his dog. But I think about them often. I do, seriously.

The next morning, I woke up and decided I was going to overdose on paracetamol and alcohol.

But first I was going to take myself along to the local pub, have one of my favourite meals from there with four pints of Heineken and *then* come home and do it.

When I came home from the pub, I saw that Rio Bravo was just starting on the television that afternoon. And minutes after that finished, The Train was on another channel. I love The Train. It reminds me of Sunday afternoons at my grandparents which is my 'happy place'. I decided I would watch Rio Bravo and The Train, finish this pack of Lucky Strike Lights and *then* I would definitely kill myself.

Forty-odd minutes into The Train there was a knock at the door, and it was a friend of mine. He was having relationship troubles and he wanted somewhere to "hide out", "depressurise from the argument" and get some advice. He chose me. I would later find out that this had all been faked for my benefit – a deliberate ruse between my friend and his partner to make me feel valued and to see that I had people who regarded me highly enough to seek advice from. But by the time he came to leave, he hugged me and thanked me and said he was lucky to have me.

I sat down on my sofa and thought to myself "Okay, maybe I <u>do</u> have friends then!"

That one thought, that one challenge of the overwhelmingly negative thought, got me thinking as to whether things really were as bleak as I was thought they were. Maybe I should look at things again now I'm a bit 'calmer'.

And that's the crux behind this anecdote you never thought was going to end; each negative thought must be weighed accurately before we allow it to press down on us. Its validity must be challenged. Because negativity is a sneaky little bitch like that. It feeds on low mood, but it *multiplies* off other negativity.

Many years later I would be receiving PTSD therapy that I found to be beneficial in many ways.

One such way was whilst I was recounting a particular negative experience and how it had left me fearful of ever taking chances in that regard again, and the therapist said to me "You are not your worst moment."

That stuck with me. I use it a lot now when helping others who are suffering with depression and other mental health issues in their day-to-day lives. Moments pass. They're replaced by other moments. Our mental ill health can become impacted when we have too many bad moments run one after the other and we think this is some sort of definition of our character, our lives, or our abilities. It isn't.

If we allow our worst moment to dictate who we are than we are not being our true selves. We're being pushed to fit the shape of something that is controlling who we see ourselves as, whilst blinding us to other important elements of truth. My God, that sounded really wanky didn't it? I vowed we weren't going to have any of that shite in this book. Let me put it *another* way – we fail an exam and then we define ourselves as a failure, without necessarily looking at the successes we had in other exams and that we were simply weaker at this one subject. Or even that we simply might not be academically minded but that we are well-skilled in other practical things or creative areas.

When I was eighteen years of age I got my A-level results. I took three and I got two A grades and a D grade. I remember coming out of school with my results to find that my mother was waiting in the car park for me. She had driven up with the intention of going in with me to receive them, missing her chance to do so by minutes.

I told her my results and she immediately responded "You got a D? Why did you even bother?" My best friend at the time replied, "But he got two A's?" only for my mum to shoot straight back "Sat alongside a D that rubs the shine off them!"

She walked back to the car, leaving me embarrassed and my friend whispering "Woah, your mum is tough going, eh?"

Because university wasn't an option for me like it was for my sister, my mum's stance carried greater weight than it probably should have.

I felt like my achievement had been diminished by that D grade, just like she said, and I didn't think I had cause to celebrate.

It wasn't until I came out the other side of my time in the military and started applying for jobs a couple of years down the line that I saw my A grade A-levels had *currency* and no one really gave two shits that I got a D grade in Sociology.

We give too much value to our failings or our weaknesses and not enough to self-recognising our assets and our significance. You don't have to be defined by the former. There is absolutely no rule, resolution, or regulation in place anywhere in the world that says you must be. We put that restriction on *ourselves*.

One of the ways we can extinguish or distance the negative thought before applying another negative thought on top - and thus create what inevitably becomes catastrophic – is by stretching the thought itself to its most incongruous and ridiculous length and looking at in that light:

Why fear leaving the house?
Because you might see someone you know!
They might see you in this state you feel you're in!
What happens if you must make small talk?
Then after making terrible small talk they go home and *die*?
You're the last person to see them alive.
The police now think you're guilty of killing this person!
All because you went out the house to buy milk...
You'llhave to go on the run like Dr Kimble in The Fugitive.
You're not going to do well at that, are you?
You're not wily in nature, you don't think well on your feet...
... And you've not done any cardio in a while.
You'll get caught quickly.
Look at the way you are right now:

You'll not present advantageously in court.
They'll 'throw the book' at you. No one will believe you.
You're going to prison. For a long time.
Best just stay home. It's scary out there.

Totally ridiculous, right? Especially written out and read back to yourself. But is that any more absurd than some of your worst thoughts in your lowest moments that you've allowed to go unchallenged? That *everyone* will turn and laugh at you in the street or something? That you're a failure at *everything*? Or that you have *no* worth at all in *any* way shape or form?

There lies the key – pour out and write down what burdens you and what your feared outcomes are that are leading you to think, see, believe things how they are. And how many of them stand as true when inarguable facts are forcibly attached to them. Let's go back to my own 'brain fart' at my lowest moment from way back when and let's stress test the shit out of that.

> My own family is actively working against me having any chance at happiness. What chance do I have at happiness when my family are championing me to fail? What is it about me that makes my own family hate me? What did I do and what do I continue to do that invites such mockery and criticism from them? Your family is meant to know you best and if they see me this way, no wonder everyone else sees me this way too. I'm just a joke to people. Everyone pushes me around and exploits me. That's why I keep struggling in work – because there's a total disconnect between how I want to be treated by people and how people think I deserve to be treated. I'm not deserved of respect. I want to be great enough at something that it almost demands respect from people, especially my family. Why can't I accept that there's great people in life and there's also-rans and I'm an also-ran? No one cares

about me. How on earth am I going to find the drive to find another job when I am inevitably just going to fuck it up and piss people off in it? If I don't find another job I'm not going to be able to keep my home. Where am I going to live? How am I going to attract a girlfriend if I don't have a job or somewhere to live? I'm not getting any younger, thinner or more attractive so why would anyone want to go out with me with all the baggage I carry? Who's going to want to marry me or have children with me? I'm just an also-ran who wishes for greatness, hated by his own family and without any friends, who's just existing rather than living and it hurts so bad each day to wake up and have to be reminded of this. If I wasn't around anymore my parents wouldn't have to keep dealing with me as an 'embarrassment'. My sister would be happy as she can go back to being the sole-focus of my parents' attention. I would finally be at peace from having to face what a loser I am. I don't have a wife or children so it isn't like there's anyone that's going to miss me anyway...

And then you go to town on it!

You systemically work through each thought, each through-line to another thought, each diversion and side-track and you put a challenge upon it. Pretend you're John McClane and you're hunting down and wiping out a terrorist, one by one and floor by floor. Like this:

1. *"My own family is actively working against me having any chance at happiness. What chance do I have at happiness when my family are championing me to fail?"*

Why is your happiness controlled by other people? Especially your family! Your chance at happiness is not in the hands of someone else and if it is take it back off them. It's not there's to have.

2. *"What is it about me that makes my own family hate me? What did I do and what do I continue to do that invites such mockery and criticism from them?"*

Why is their mockery and criticism valid? Ask them! Challenge them. If your family really do hate you because you're not living up to their expectations that is a pretty pitiful reflection on them. Why put their issues on you?

3. *"Your family is meant to know you best and if they see me this way, no wonder everyone else sees me this way too."*

Who is everyone? That's really generalised. How do you know they see you the same way? Why do you assume your family know you best? Because they spent the most amount of time with you when you were a child? You're an adult now. You spend more time in the company of other people than them.

4. *"I'm just a joke to people."*

Again, this is generalised. What people? List them all up. Push yourself to name who. And in what way. If you work with ten people, then exhibit the evidence that all ten think of you as a joke.

5. *"Everyone pushes me around and exploits me."*

In what way? Exemplify it. Why let them? Who says you must endure that? What ways could you better challenge it in a healthy and productive way.

6. *"That's why I keep struggling in work – because there's a total disconnect between how I want to be treated by people and how people think I deserve to be treated. I'm not deserved of respect."*

Why are you not deserved of respect? How have you come to this rationalisation or line of thought? There may be an issue around you receiving a level of respect in your personal or professional life but where is the evidence that you're not deserved of any?

7. *"I want to be great enough at something that it almost demands respect from people, especially my family. Why can't I accept that there's great people in life and there's also-rans and I'm an also-ran?"*

Achieving greatness as a means of achieving emotional validation can be pretty empty 'greatness' and may not lead where you think. Who says you're an 'also-ran'? You? On what basis?

8. *"No one cares about me."*

No one? No one at all? Look around you at the friends who rally when you sink low or the family member who takes two forms of public transport just to come and check on you, the stranger and his dog who stop to talk because they sense you could do with a human connection? These things may seem small against the weight of other feelings, but they matter. Be careful not to confuse a generalisation with a major fact.

9. *"How on earth am I going to find the drive to find another job when I am inevitably just going to fuck it up and piss people off in it?"*

How are you going to fuck it up? You don't even have it yet. You don't know what it is, where it is or what it is doing to know whether you can! You're projecting a fear and taking it as an actuality.

10. *"If I don't find another job I'm not going to be able to keep my home. Where am I going to live?"*

What evidence is there that you're at a stage where you're going to lose your home? Is this a reality or catastrophic thinking that you're allowing to dominate?

11. *"How am I going to attract a girlfriend if I don't have a job or somewhere to live?"* and *"I'm not getting any younger, thinner or more attractive so why would anyone want to go out with me with all the baggage I carry?"*

Is this the right priority for right now? Even if you want to pursue it as a line of thought for this moment over concentrating on yourself, you have no knowledge of what every single woman finds attractive in every single man. You don't know what one person goes for in a partner. Look at Eva Braun.

12. *"Who's going to want to marry me or have children with me?"*

Are you looking to marry or enter parenthood next week? No? Then calm down. You don't know what's round the corner.

13. *"I'm just an also-ran who wishes for greatness, hated by his own family and without any friends, who's just existing rather than living and it hurts so bad each day to wake up and have to be reminded of this."*

Go back to the also-ran stuff and push harder down on it. Your life isn't over. No one has come and pressed 'stop' on you. Who says you must stand still in this feeling and this moment and have your life defined by how you're feeling right now? What rule says you must do that?

14. *"If I wasn't around anymore my parents wouldn't have to keep dealing with me as an 'embarrassment'. My sister would be happy as she can go back to being the sole-focus of my parents' attention."*

Hey, if you weren't around anymore your parents would inevitably have to suffer the quiet judgment of others because there's always someone out there that'll look on them as having 'failed' you and it sounds to me that by 'sticking around' you're pissing your sibling off and that sounds like a good enough reason as any to me.

15. *"I would finally be at peace from having to face what a loser I am."*

Who says you're a loser? What's so great about them that means they get to label and define you? What makes you a loser? List the reasons. For every reason you must provide tangible, actual evidence alongside it.

16. *"I don't have a wife or children so it isn't like there's anyone that's going to miss me anyway..."*

You don't need a wife and a child to be missed. You have friends, we've established that. You don't know what individual and personal impact your existence has on those around you, and you can't possibly know in absolute certainty therefore what you're saying can't be a fact.

Your own will be <u>very</u> different in the detail, obviously.

But once you've done that you can see that you have a lot of thoughts that don't stand up on their own.

Think of it as if you're putting a file of evidence together to go before the court.

It must be complete, with all facts of the case gathered. There is very little chance of that case succeeding with a whole heap of unanswered questions in the air that could support the defence. So, what we do here is we take our 'file', and we omit all of the stuff that isn't holding up to scrutiny as is and needs further evidence applied. We look at what we're left with after that and we judge how strong a case we have then.

We go back over what our catastrophised thought is and we strip away all the assumptions, the generalisations, and the things we don't know with the utmost certainty to be true.

Like this:

> ~~My own family is actively working against me having any chance at happiness. What chance do I have at happiness when my family are championing me to fail? What is it about me that makes my own family hate me? What did I do and what do I continue to do that invites such mockery and criticism from them? Your family is meant to know you best and if they see me this way, no wonder everyone else sees me this way too. I'm just a joke to people. Everyone pushes me around and exploits me. That's why I keep struggling in work – because~~ there's a total disconnect between how I want to be treated by people and how people think I deserve to be treated. ~~I'm not deserved of respect. I want to be great enough at something that it almost demands respect from people, especially my family. Why can't I accept that there's great people in life and there's also-rans and I'm an also-ran? No one cares about me. How on earth am I going to find the drive to find another job when I am inevitably just going to fuck it up and piss people off in it? If I don't find another job I'm not going to be able to keep my home. Where am I going to live? How am I going to attract a girlfriend if I don't have a job or somewhere to live?~~ I'm not getting any younger, ~~thinner or more attractive~~

~~so why would anyone want to go out with me with all the baggage I carry? Who's going to want to marry me or have children with me? I'm just an also-ran who wishes for greatness, hated by his own family and without any friends, who's just existing rather than living and it hurts so bad each day to wake up and have to be reminded of this. If I wasn't around anymore my parents wouldn't have to keep dealing with me as an 'embarrassment'. My sister would be happy as she can go back to being the sole-focus of my parents' attention. I would finally be at peace from having to face what a loser I am. I don't have a wife or children so it isn't like there's anyone that's going to miss me anyway...~~

What are we left with?

You could argue that this disconnect between how you want to be treated and how you feel you're treated is worth exploring, were it not for the fact that you're projecting the notion that you know what people "think" in this scenario.

Objectively though what you're *actually* left with is:

I'm not getting any younger.

That's the fact. Amongst all the catastrophic thinking we looked at there, it is the only fact.

Give it a try for yourself.

To part-quote the poet laureate that is Taylor Swift;

"... Got a long list of ex-lovers.
They'll tell you I'm insane.
But I've got a blank space, baby..."

I will end this chapter with this though:

Sometimes when I'm in a low mood and I desperately want to find something to ward it off before it develops into a worsening state of mind, I think back to that man and his dog Oliver, late on a cold January night in 2008. I think back to them and I'm quietly thankful for them because I know they saved my life and by doing so I got to experience a life further down the line that has my children in it.

"I Feel Seen" #2

MIDNIGHT RUN

Midnight Run was a film that I'd first experienced in my late teens, and it made only the mildest of impressions. I now regard it as my favourite film. Of all time. The proverbial flag that sits atop of thousands of others. Around that time, I'd spend every Friday night at my paternal grandfather's house. He'd been diagnosed with lung cancer on top of the leukaemia he already had, and he'd only been given about 6 months to live. He'd hang on in for another two years on top of that. And he fuckin **hated** that this was the case. "Waiting to die" was just not for him.

Every Friday night I'd get on my bike, ride over to his, get all his medications aligned, change bedsheets, mow his lawn every three or four weeks per visit, pick up the money for a video rental and our fish and chips then head back out to the shops round the corner. His frequent instruction for film choice was always only "Blood and boobs!" He was mostly deaf at this stage and hated wearing hearing aids inside of the house, so he liked his films with little talking, lots of action and violence and for a bit of a female nudity. No prolonged "sexiness" though. It made him uncomfortable in all the ways you would assume it to, watching it with your grandson.

Together we'd watch some of the best and worst of straight-to-video action films of the late eighties and early nineties.

Midnight Run was a blind rental on the video shop owner's recommendation.

Because the one my grandad had sent me in to get was out and there was such a dearth of alternative options.

The one that he sent me to get was Men of War, starring Dolph Lundgren – and written by no less than the legendary John Sayles! The fact that I remember this very clear three decades later definitely makes me think I'm somewhere on the neurodivergent scale, seeing as my memory for things of actual use is terrible.

I went with it, we watched it together and, back then, at seventeen, I thought it was *okay* – funny, some good action sequences and what not. My grandad didn't like it because there was too much talking and not enough action.

Flash forward nearly eight years and I was a hard-drinking depressive, scraping a living as a Civil Servant in a role I detested and burnt-out from my military experience and getting ran out of a job thereafter for standing up against wrongdoing. In the process of all that happening I'd gotten stabbed, saw my still-undiagnosed PTSD worsen as a result and landed back in the same city as my parents who told me once again what an embarrassment I was proving.

"Have you ever asked yourself what it is about you that makes people hate you as much they do?" asked my sister around this time. "Because your mum and dad and I have a life we're very happy in and you keep dropping back into it after getting kicked to the gutter by another job and another group of friends who've stabbed you in the back, expecting us to pull you back up on to your feet and that's not fair on us. We don't deserve to have to carry the shame of you keep messing your life up."

My parents sat nodding sagely in agreement as she spoke.

That night I went on a disastrous night out down the coast, drinking with my then-girlfriend and her circle of friends. I caught her cheating on me out the back of a bar, much to her friends' amusement, I confronted them both and got summarily beaten up by the guy she was cheating on me with. I ended up with a broken nose for the third of four times as a result.

I staggered home alone, put a bag of frozen sweetcorn on my face and crashed down in front of BBC1.

With a full packet of cigarettes, nobody to have to interact with and half a bottle of Jim Beam in front of me the possibility of the night being rescued was looking like a real possibility.

I found Midnight Run showing as a late night movie - with all the swearing dubbed out, and anyone who knows this film well knows how horrifying that is. Because this is a film that makes ***art*** out of the word "fuck".

It was the character backstory that stood out to me this time round. It hit me and it resonated *hard* - Jack Walsh (Robert De Niro) is a tough ex-cop who used to work the streets of Chicago. Plot exposition reveals that whilst working undercover to capture a psychotic heroin dealer called Jimmy Serrano (Dennis Farina), Walsh's cover is blown, and he is left exposed by the corrupt officers in his precinct. Walsh tries to expose the corruption in the Chicago PD but Serrano and the cops on his payroll chase him down and force him to quit. With that backstory out of the way, the film begins several years later:

Serrano is now one of the biggest mob bosses on the west coast. Walsh is now a bum, estranged from his wife and daughter and scraping a living as a bounty hunter for foul-mouthed bail bondsman Eddie Moscone (Joe Pantoliano). He wants out of this life and is offered $100,000 for an easy gig, a 'midnight run', if he can find a fugitive called Jonathan 'The Duke' Mardukas (Charles Grodin) and bring him into LA alive, before the bail bond is null and void subsequently bankrupting Moscone. The hook? Mardukas was working as a mob bookkeeper and embezzled $15 million of Serrano's money. Once in custody he has the means to bring Walsh's arch-nemesis down once and for all. But standing in Jack Walsh's way is the FBI, Serrano's hitmen and Mardukas himself, who will do everything he can to outwit Walsh and escape from his custody.

I watched this film, laughed through the pain in places and genuinely didn't think about my swollen face or the humiliation I'd just suffered for the whole of its running time.

I just kept looking at the character of Jack Walsh and muttering drunkenly to myself about how I'd spoken out about corruption too, how I'd been kicked to the curb, how I was a bum working shit-house jobs I didn't really want but had to make a living.

'The Duke':
"There's good and bad everywhere, don't you think?"

Jack Walsh:
"Well, I'd say there's bad everywhere. Good, I don't know about!"

The next morning with a painful nose and a stinking hangover, I could not get the film out of my mind. It wasn't running entirely clearly through my head, but I could remember laughing with it and being on the edge of my seat in places and bouncing along to an infectious musical score.

Most importantly I remember crying at the end and feeling... *something*. Something that was lingering on the next day, making me think about not wanting to feel the way I'd been feeling or live how I'd been living.

I took a walk down to my local fleapit video store and found it in a video tape bargain basket in the corner of the shop. I snapped it up and rushed home. I watched Midnight Run twice that afternoon back to back.

What really seals the film as one of the greatest action comedies on top of the wonderfully played friendship that we watch form between DeNiro's Walsh and Grodin's Mardukas, is the little background characters!

In your normal run of the mill movie of this type these would be people that you would not give a second glance to.

But in Midnight Run even the minor characters are given little traits to help them shine that little bit brighter.

And the film is all the better for it; from Mosley's assistants bickering amongst each other because one has a chronic ability to say exactly the wrong thing at the wrong time, through to Tony and Joey, Serrano's two incompetent henchmen who don't let the task their boss has assigned them get in the way of just having fun.

(There's a brilliant little scene where they ring back their boss to let him know they have failed and Walsh/Mardukas are alive and have escaped. Whilst Serrano berates them and threatens them down the phone, they quietly play fight with each other as he does this).

The film is a thoroughly engaging one despite its action genre status. The characters are so real that you feel as if they really did exist, outside of the confines of the film's running time before the film started and will exist long after the film has ended (although the misjudged TV movies in the mid-90s with Christopher Macdonald as Walsh don't do well in backing up this fact).

Jack Walsh suddenly became my 'spirit guide' for the years that came thereafter. I'll never be able to fully articulate *exactly* what it was about the character that impacted me so severely in that moment, but I saw so much of myself in him, just like I had with Dawn Wiener in Welcome To The Dollhouse. I drew from his stoic resilience in the face of all the indignities and injustices that had been bestowed upon him, I admired his sense of righteousness and the code he sort of lived by.

That evening, I packed up my girlfriend's things and placed them in the hallway. I threw away the bottles of spirits that took up an entire cupboard in the kitchen. And I vowed to try and be *better*.

Had I not done so in that moment I would not have ended up going down the more improved path in life that I did, which was a path that *eventually* led me to my wife and my beloved children.

Midnight Run made me do that.

"I Wasn't Aiming For You!"

Goals, Targets, Etc.

The funniest thing one of my closest friends ever confided in me – and which I have his hesitant permission to share with you anecdotally here – is that the search engines on his online porn history now veer towards the 'older' lady. He's in his early forties now, so that should give you a frame of reference as to what we mean by '*older*'. He explained that since he was a teenager his fantasy has always involved the older 'MILF' type and that's never changed, he's just got older himself. (You can pretend you don't know what 'MILF' means all you like, but you'll be looking up its meaning in your *own* time!), He reasoned that if he was ageing than it made perfect sense to him that his 'tastes' would age to.

Now, as funny as his 'take' is in terms of the whole "whatever turns you on" thing (and if my dear Grandmother was still around, I certainly wouldn't be leaving him alone with her), there is something earnest to draw from his stance: Our goals should be individual to us and remain flexible and adjustable given other impacting factors... I bet that's not where you thought this *particular yarn* was going to end up, did you?

A whole 'other lifetime' ago I used to do a bit of boxing.

We can talk more about that later.

I remember training as part of a team for a particular competition and it was my first time competing at this sort of level, as well as training in this sort of charged and very 'alpha' environment.

I had been a 'reserve' on the team up until this point, and I was being called on last minute to fill a slot taken by a middleweight who'd suffered an injury.

I was used to just coming into the gym when most people were gone and kind of phoning it in but here, I was having to skip alongside others, do heavy bag work side by side with people who hit harder and faster than I did, and I would frequently get very self-conscious and distracted by how good everyone else was compared to me. One day my coach caught me staring at a huge heavyweight pounding on a bag repeatedly, indenting it with force I was far from capable of doing and he slapped me on the back of the head. "What are you looking at what he's doing for?" he barked. "He's training for a different fight to you!"

And he was right. In many ways in life overall, aren't we all? That guy's training was specific to the challenge ahead that *he* was facing. It was focusing on accentuating his strengths and improving his weaknesses. Not mine. Too often when we're setting ourselves goals or targets, we're getting too focused on outside 'noise' and ancillary people, comparing ourselves to them or setting ourselves an outcome of wanting to better *them* or earn respect from them. I wasted so many years of my life, absent of any self-esteem, setting myself goals and objectives that were designed to make *other people* happy or to fulfil a plan or an agenda *they* had.

We set goals to make changes, adjustments and improvements in our lives because doing so helps increase the motivation needed to affect the change we want to see or feel. We can use them to improve relationships, sure. But they must be <u>our</u> goals and we must be very careful not to allow another person's agenda or wishes to infect or ultimately become ours. If you set your goal at losing weight, for example, and you're doing so because you want to impress a prospective partner than the goal will falter and fail should you find that said potential partner isn't interested in you, regardless of your size. But if you set your weight-loss target around improving your health, your physicality, and your feeling of self-worth it is far easier to stay on track and acquire someone who finds you attractive along the way.

There's that cliché you see in old westerns or action movies where the hero fires a shot past the villain and the villain exclaims "You missed!" and the protagonist replies "I wasn't aiming for you!" or something akin to that, and you see that he was actually shooting out the support beam of something for it to fall on the villains head or a nearby fuse wire that then blows up the barrel of gunpowder.

You get what I am referring to, right?

I used to watch Transformers: Prime with my youngest son. There's a bit in it where Optimus Prime shoots towards Dreadwing and Dreadwing cackles "Your aim is poor!" Then the glacier behind Dreadwing starts to crack from the gunshot and Prime replies "That is a matter of perspective!" and the glacier crumbles into an avalanche and Dreadwing gets buried.

The point is you aim for what you need to aim for. Don't let anybody else tell you what that needs to be. At the heaviest weight of the depression sitting on your chest and making it feel like you can't breathe the number one most unhelpful thing to hear in the world is someone saying, "You just need to pull yourself together, man." In that state of mind 'pulling yourself together' feels so huge and unreachable. Why not aim for just getting out of bed and spending some time in a different room? Who's to say that this isn't good enough?

Whoever it is – *fuck 'em*!

For example, you can look over to that person at the gym who is chest pressing 150kg and bemoan that you can't do that and that makes you lesser than them. Or you can acknowledge that the person currently chest pressing 150kg once started out at 20kg and slowly, incrementally moved the weight up with consistent effort over time. You don't need to find comfort in lifting what *they're* lifting. It's too heavy for where you're at. You need to lift what *you're* comfortable with and move upwards from there. There are metaphors for and analogies to mental health tucked away in that example, don't you think?

Make your goal setting, certainly specific to your fight against mental ill health, like a three-course meal; begin with a small 'starter', lead towards a 'main course' and finish with a 'dessert' that pays off nicely against what you've "eaten" up to that point.

It burns me a little to admit this because I wish I was clever enough to devise something so much better and more useful, but the truth is I vowed that throughout this book I would put forward to you the things that worked for me and when it comes to setting myself goals or targets around my mental health or the improvement of my emotional well-being I've not yet found a better way of structuring and tracking it then the SMART method.

Yeah, that's right – remember that thing they used to teach us in school and pushed hard on us as a way of setting targets and achieving them? Well, it turns out that unlike some things they taught us in school that they said were important (how often are *you* using algebra in your day-to-day life, huh?), this is "too legit to quit" as the three-time Grammy Award / eight-time American Music Award / People's Choice / Billboard Diamond Award winning artiste MC Hammer once said. ("*... Cause you don't want none, I hustle for my muscle and you look weak, son...*")

In case you've forgotten, or you weren't paying attention at school the SMART method is designed to make goal or target setting feel tangible and within your grasp. It stands for **S**pecific, **M**easurable, **A**chievable, **R**elevant and **T**ime-Based. As in you clearly define what it is you want to attain (specific), you add marker indicators in some way or form to be able to track your progress (measurable), make certain that what you're targeting is realistic (achievable), ensure the goal you're setting yourself is reflective of a wider ambition or drive for yourself (relevant) and that you have a deadline you can hold yourself to in order to maintain focus (time-based).

It will really seem silly to some of you to sit down with a notepad and pen or an open notes screen on your phone and do something like this but you'll be very surprised how effective it can be.

By being clear with yourself about what it is you want to achieve, you become more focused on where you need to concentrate your efforts and by starting small you can use the success of one goal as the foundation for another. For me personally, I found setting goals using this method and keeping track of them a great way of identifying at what points I was getting distracted or waylaid in pursuit of the goal (especially around diet and exercise) and then I could refine or adjust the SMART target and go again with a greater chance of success. If your target is to eat healthily for a week, for example, and you fail four days in because you binged on a packet of biscuits then you know to not have tempting things in the house, omit them from the next week's shop, re-set the target and go again.

Ultimately, we do this, and we track it because (let's be frank here) the "doing" is a grind and often it may not feel enjoyable but it's the smaller requirement to work through to achieve the greater end result. So, we monitor the progress to *own* that achievement along the way, which goes someway to working on your self-esteem and your confidence... which in turn gets those neurotransmitters sending all the 'good shit' out from 'Central HQ' (also biologically known as your brain).

The key lies in looking at the bigger picture of where you want to be long term and funneling that all the way down to a really small starting point.

A starting point where success at the start will lead to you setting yourself a renewed goal a little bit more ambitious than the next...

... and the next...

... and so on, until each completed goal has widened out and you're on track to be where you want to be.

Think of it like a computer game where the level starts out with you beating up progressively more difficult bad guys until you get to the 'big boss'. I think we've done enough already for you to be applying your own Die Hard points of reference at this stage, yes?

Or a reverse pyramid.

Think of it as a reverse pyramid.

(Mainly because I've already got the point illustrated with a pyramid to use imminently, not a computer game. Sorry.)

Exercise is a very easy one to use as an example but don't think this is what you must lead with. We're going to talk about exercise later in the book but when it comes to goal setting the only thing you must keep in mind is that it is intrinsically individual to you and that you must always start small.

If you're off work sick and it is related to mental health problems than your depression could be affecting your sleep, your appetite, and your state of mind. Studies have shown even now people off sick with stress and anxiety related illnesses or impactors still tend to isolate themselves away and avoid leaving the house to see friends or complete tasks because they have a fear they'll be 'spotted' by a colleague or their boss when they are out and accused of fraudulent sickness.

It's a fallacy to believe that because you are suffering from acute stress which leaves you unable to work you cannot therefore leave the house. Most GPs, talking therapists, etc will actively *encourage* you to get out / see friends and exercise. If you're in a position akin to this then your starting goal is going to be getting dressed, then leaving the house, seeing friends, getting comfortable in social situations again, beginning a phased return to work and then eventually being back at work full time again.

Setting goals is a means to help you consider and assess what you want to achieve or work towards in your life which means that the goals can be wide-ranging across a variety of areas in your life. They can be educational or in the field of continued professional development, they can therefore also be career-orientated and financial, familial, physical, or emotional. They can even be simply artistic or for pleasure.

One friend of mine had no musical abilities with instruments or had even shown a curiosity in that regard.

He picked up an interest in a specific type of electronic dance music and decided to set himself a goal of learning how that music is made and releasing a track of his own creation all within just one year. And that friend you might now know as a DJ called *Skrillex*.

Just kidding. It totally wasn't.

But my friend achieved that goal. Now, I listen to the core four 'corners' of music (Journey, Air Supply, Starship and Bon Jovi) with the occasional daytrip into 'fancy stuff' (Chicago, Sister Hazel and Dave Grusin's soundtrack to the major motion picture, Tootsie); my friend's music is "not quite my tempo" to say the least. But regardless, how impressive is his achievement?

For ease though, let's put our aforementioned reverse pyramid within the broadest example of an exercise related goal so you can see in a more generalised way the level at which we *pace* our goals.

Run a half marathon.

Be able to run 10 miles.

Be able run 5 miles.

Be able to run 3 miles.

Be able to run 1 mile.

Walk 101 steps daily.

Walk 3 times a week.

Leave the house.

Breathe.

Once you've decided on what that 'starter' goal is, you've got to keep on top of it and that's going to require you reviewing it regularly, carrying out that self-inventory and holding yourself to account. If your goal is to force yourself up out of bed every day and take a shower then set a little note screen up on your phone with a tick box next to every day of the week, throw a tick in the box the minute you step out of the shower. If the SMART target was just you getting out of bed every day that week and taking a shower than... *BAM!* ... Congratulations, you've nailed it!

And make the goals positive, yeah?

Trust me from experience here, there's no point filling up notes on your phone's relevant app with shit like "Stop fucking up!" or "Be more tolerable to people!" They don't fit into the SMART model, do they? They're just reinforcing a line of thinking that doesn't hold up to fact-checking like we discussed in an earlier chapter. It's all just 'noise' that reinforces a negative mind-set. You're going to nail these goals once you get going and the goals themselves expand so why get distracted or slowed down with things and thoughts that are only going to hamper your progress?

Let's finish on a couple of examples of SMART goals that have been helpful to me in terms of working on impactors around my mental health:

I want to lose weight because I have stopped going out so much lately due to feeling self-conscious about my physical appearance.

Specific	I am going to lose a minimum of 13lbs in 6 weeks by eating healthily under my calorie level for my weight, age, and height.
Measurable	I am going to use a calorie-tracking app like MyFitnessPal to record what I am eating each day and that it is within my calorie limit.
Attainable	This is realistic and attainable because if I consider what I eat and remain in a calorie deficit than I will lose weight. I have also set myself a target time wise that is not unrealistic.
Relevant	The goal is relevant because I want to lose weight to improve my feelings of self-worth, and this is an effective way of doing that.
Time-Based	I have set a target of 6 weeks and will monitor whether it needs altered slightly depending on weight loss in the first four weeks.

By checking regularly on how you're getting on and keeping a record, no matter how small, you can take a goal like this and off-set a chance of failure.

For example, you're tracking your weight, and you can see that there was a huge immediate loss in the first week of 4lbs but you've lost only 1lb a week every week thereafter. It's now Week 5 and you have lost 8lbs but this is only just passed halfway on the way to your goal, with one week to go by your initial draft.

You don't hand-grenade the whole effort.

You don't quit.

You simply *recalibrate.*

You go back to your SMART goal, and you adjust the time element by another two, three or four weeks and then you carry on.

I want to improve my relationships with my friends over the course of the next month as I have allowed my mental health to affect my interactions with them.

Specific	I am going to contact a minimum of two friends and maintain regular contact with them, responding in a timely manner to their texts or calls.
Measurable	This is realistically measurable because the level and flow of contact and time distances between responses will be recorded on my phone's call and message logs as evidence for me to check..
Attainable	This is realistic because it is a low number of people and the pressure is low in terms of communication, not

	necessarily social outings at this point.
Relevant	It's relevant because if I don't try with my friends than they will lose interest in making an effort with me and there won't be a means to maintain the friendship.
Time-Based	I have set a target of over the course of one month so consistency of communication can be achieved and hopefully set as a new standard to move forward with.

The first time you sit down and start formulating this, I assure you that you're going to feel a bit self-conscious and a little silly. The thing is though there's a reason there's a whole multimillion dollar 'speaker circuit' industry out there, exploiting vulnerable folk with trussed up and overcomplicated versions of pyramid-related SMART target 'speak'.

It's because at its most simplified core it *works*.

And that's reflected in the fact that if you stop and scrutinise yourself in your day to day life as is, at work, with jobs around the house or in your child's development... you're passively doing some variation of it *anyway* as a natural mental process. Here all you're doing is recording it and keeping a trail of it to help yourself out a little better.

The 'Compartmentalisation of Time' Method

Having worked out your goals, you've just got to find the time to get going with them – right? And don't say you *don't* have time. Don't lie to yourself like that. You could say you're not that good at making time to go after your goals, though this chapter will hopefully change that. But don't say the time isn't there, available to you. Do you have any idea how much your depression, anxiety, stress, etc *steals* from you outright when you are at your weakest, and it is in control of you instead of the other way round? You know that boxset of whatever season of television you're zoned out in front of under your blanket whilst hiding away from the world? Have you looked at the running time on *that*?

At (one of) the peak points of a bad depressive episode in my late twenties I once sat and watched every single John Carpenter movie back-to-back. In one sitting. Not including his TV movies (Someone's Watching Me, Elvis and Body Bags) or The Ward (because he hadn't made that yet). But quite literally back-to-back, in one position with just breaks for the toilet or to top up my drinks. Now, I'm not going to lie to you, it was a lot of fun because John Carpenter movies are predominantly frickin' *awesome* (and short; his longest movie is Starman at a relatively breezy 115 minutes) but it was neither healthy nor responsible.

I woke up one day and found myself unable to face what was ahead of me 'outside', I cancelled the plans and obligations I had, and I looked for a route to 'escape'. This was it.

I started with 1974's Dark Star (83 minutes) and I finished with Ghost of Mars (96 minutes).

In between I watched 16 films (including the first sequel to Halloween that *everyone knows* he secretly reshot and recalibrated because Rick Rosenthal made a disaster of it), one after the other after the other with my phone switched off and the door locked.

I shut out the outside world and most of my negative thoughts for 1,569 minutes straight. That's just over 26 hours. Did it help me in that moment? I kidded myself that it did. But did it help me long-term or move me forward. I took the [*correct*] notion that movies can 'help' and I went too far in the wrong direction at the cost of showing up for my friend's birthday meal or going round to visit my grandma.

Could I have watched a John Carpenter movie at a rate of one a night, every night as a little treat to myself to help my mood and sort of reward myself after a day of surviving / enduring / working towards my goal(s) or on my mental health? *Absolutely*. But that's if I was in control. I wasn't. My ill health was.

My mental health was dictating my schedule and setting my diary and that was never going to work out well because the thing with depression is that it doesn't want you to do anything but think negatively because negative thinking breeds negative thoughts.

Depression and the like must be very careful about letting you do *anything* because that *anything* might turn into *something* that helps you combat it – and it <u>can't</u> have that. So, it needs to keep you away from the things, the people and the places that could generate positivity, hope and all that 'nice shit'.

There's a whole heap of folk out there that 'sell' time management as some sort of taught 'skill' when it really doesn't need to be looked at like that at all.

Arnold Schwarzenegger has a <u>great</u> approach to looking at how you spend and utilise your time, and he's frequently giving it away *for free* on his social media platforms:

It's common-sense stuff that relates to how you look personally at the value of your time, not any sort of 'science' around the manipulation or the quantitive reinterpretation of it.

It's about what you do with the time you have not time itself.

Or to put it another way, it's about what you put inside of the bag more than it is about the colour of the bag. My method is called 'The Compartmentalisation of Time'. One, because it sounds 'fancy' and two, the whole process relates to categorising your time into controlled blocks that you hold ownership of.

To get going, you've got to initially admit to yourself in the first instance that when your mental health is controlling you, as opposed to the other way round, your time is not being used effectively. It is being controlled by a negative state of mind that is just absolutely *pissing away* your time.

If you were to start out by logging your days activities and then looking back over them, you'd probably see a whole heap of 'dead time' that you've just allowed to eke out once you got trapped in a line of negative thinking.

When I'm planning my time – and when you're starting out on this journey towards taking back control of your mental health this is something you <u>must</u> do – I work in two hour blocks. If you were to go off the notion of a working day, plus the average amount of recommended sleep, a **bad** day would look something like this:

00:00 – 02:00	Try to get to sleep.
02:00 – 04:00	Sleep.
04:00 – 06:00	Sleep.
06:00 – 08:00	Sleep / Get up / Get washed / Get ready for work / Breakfast.
08:00 – 10:00	Travel to work / Work.

10:00 – 12:00	Work.
12:00 – 14:00	Lunch / Work.
14:00 – 16:00	Work.
16:00 – 18:00	Work / Travel home.
18:00 – 20:00	Sit at home alone / Eat / Wash / Watch TV
20:00 – 22:00	Watch TV
22:00 – 00:00	Watch TV / Try to get to sleep.

But we're setting goals, and we need time to *work* on those goals, as well as unwind from the day and fulfil our obligations like work and sleep.

(We all know what this same schedule would look like if we are unemployed or off work for mental health reasons. Don't tell me that we wouldn't be seeing the same Breaking Bad, Sopranos, Band of Brothers boxset or streamed medical drama on repeat mention here.)

So, we look at the day and we review it for what I call 'stealable time'. This is time you can claim back and do what you want with. On review, it should look something like this:

00:00 – 02:00	Try to get to sleep.
02:00 – 04:00	Sleep.
04:00 – 06:00	Sleep.
06:00 – 08:00	Sleep / Get up / Get washed / Get ready for work / Breakfast.
08:00 – 10:00	Travel to work / Work.
10:00 – 12:00	Work.
12:00 – 14:00	Lunch / Work.
14:00 – 16:00	Work.
16:00 – 18:00	Work / Travel home.

18:00 – 20:00	Sit at home alone / Eat / Wash / Watch TV
20:00 – 22:00	Watch TV
22:00 – 00:00	Watch TV / Try to get to sleep.

We're looking at five compartments of time that equate to approximately ten hours in a twenty-four hour day.

All those thoughts of "I'd love to learn a new language and get fit and see my friends more often, but I just don't have the time. There are not enough hours in the day." Well guess what? You've just been given ten hours back that were hidden away within you all along.

Now we're going to create an itinerary for ourselves moving forward and we're going to get ourselves a couple of highlighter pens (if you're old school) or some nice pastel tabs on your phone's notepad (if you're technically minded) and we're going to create our 'dream' schedule to incorporate our SMART goal(s).

00:00 – 02:00	Try to get to sleep.
02:00 – 04:00	Sleep.
04:00 – 06:00	Sleep.
06:00 – 08:00	Get up / Get washed / Get ready for work / Breakfast.
08:00 – 10:00	Travel to work / Work.
10:00 – 12:00	Work.
12:00 – 14:00	Lunch (Read a book specific to my SMART goal) / Work.
14:00 – 16:00	Work.
16:00 – 18:00	Work / Go to the gym.
18:00 – 20:00	Exercise
20:00 – 22:00	Come home / Eat / Wash / Watch TV
22:00 – 00:00	Read a book specific to my SMART goal / Try to get to sleep.

Colour code them accordingly if you're at a point where you're 'maintaining' a completed goal whilst working on a new one. And if you're one of those who's wondering why there's not a colour coded example here, let me just rant at you for a bit about how much it costs to get a book printed with colour pages nowadays!

00:00 – 02:00	Try to get to sleep.
02:00 – 04:00	Sleep.
04:00 – 06:00	Sleep / Get up / Get washed / Get ready for work.
06:00 – 08:00	Breakfast / Work on my SMART goal.
08:00 – 10:00	Travel to work / Work.
10:00 – 12:00	Work.
12:00 – 14:00	Lunch (Read a book specific to my SMART goal) / Work.
14:00 – 16:00	Work.
16:00 – 18:00	Work / Go to the gym.
18:00 – 20:00	Exercise.
20:00 – 22:00	Go out to see friends / Have a meal
22:00 – 00:00	Come home / Try to get to sleep.

You must remember that the scheduling relates to your goals because the work on or around these goals, the journaling and the tracking is all the little steps that put distance between you and the negative aspects of your mental health that control your day if you allow them to. But the goals are wholly individual to you, and you must start small.

The size needs to be comparable against what you feel you can manage. Remember how I talked earlier about your fight being different to the fight the guy next to you is facing?

Well, both your "training schedules" will be different too.

So, if you're off work because of your mental health and your day looks like this as standard:

00:00 – 02:00	Sit awake, thinking.
02:00 – 04:00	Sit awake, thinking.
04:00 – 06:00	Sleep.
06:00 – 08:00	Sleep.
08:00 – 10:00	Sleep.
10:00 – 12:00	Get up / watch TV.
12:00 – 14:00	Watch TV.
14:00 – 16:00	Watch TV.
16:00 – 18:00	Watch TV.
18:00 – 20:00	Watch TV.
20:00 – 22:00	Watch TV.
22:00 – 00:00	Watch TV.

… then your revised schedule looks like this to start out with:

00:00 – 02:00	Sit awake, thinking.
02:00 – 04:00	Sit awake, thinking.
04:00 – 06:00	Sleep.
06:00 – 08:00	Sleep.
08:00 – 10:00	Sleep.
10:00 – 12:00	Get up / Shower / watch TV.
12:00 – 14:00	Watch TV.
14:00 – 16:00	Go for a walk.
16:00 – 18:00	Watch TV.
18:00 – 20:00	Watch TV.
20:00 – 22:00	Watch TV.
22:00 – 00:00	Watch TV.

... because it may well be that where you're at right now your mental health 'owns' twenty-four hours of your day. Who's to say you can't have a couple of hours back? Who's going to miss a couple of hours?

Then... well... then we 'steal' a little more:

00:00 – 02:00	Sit awake, thinking.
02:00 – 04:00	Sit awake, thinking.
04:00 – 06:00	Sleep.
06:00 – 08:00	Sleep.
08:00 – 10:00	Sleep.
10:00 – 12:00	Get up / Shower / Watch TV.
12:00 – 14:00	Watch TV.
14:00 – 16:00	Go for a walk.
16:00 – 18:00	Watch TV.
18:00 – 20:00	Call a friend for a chat.
20:00 – 22:00	Watch TV.
22:00 – 00:00	Watch TV.

Eventually you'll come to associate a colour with a 'thing' as you gain greater control over your mental health and your goals.

And you'll come to really find value in what works at helping you, what you enjoy and before you know it you have a weekend coming up and you start to compartmentalise what that 'ideal' day looks like and all of a sudden you've jigsaw-pieced together the sort of day full of things that nourish you in a way where you've put some distance between you and the things that *don't* nourish or fulfil you.

00:00 – 02:00	Sleep.

02:00 – 04:00	Sleep.
04:00 – 06:00	Sleep.
06:00 – 08:00	Sleep.
08:00 – 10:00	Get up / Go to gym.
10:00 – 12:00	Exercise.
12:00 – 14:00	Lunch / Family activity / Family walk.
14:00 – 16:00	Family activity / Family walk.
16:00 – 18:00	Family activity / Family walk.
18:00 – 20:00	Meal out and drinks with partner and/or friends.
20:00 – 22:00	Meal out and drinks with partner and/or friends.
22:00 – 00:00	Come home / Watch a film.

Here's two blank tables for you.

Use the first to reflect over the day you've just had, fill it out and then review it to identify the 'stealable time'.

What are you looking at?

A whole lot or not much?

Now in the second one, construct and compartmentalise what your day would look like with 'total control'. To do this fill in the compartments where your obligations are fixed – your working hours, how much sleep you generally allocate yourself, any carer responsibilities. With the compartments that are empty what are you going to put in them?

What are you not doing now that you would like to?

Write 'em in there!

Present:

00:00 – 02:00	
02:00 – 04:00	
04:00 – 06:00	
06:00 – 08:00	
08:00 – 10:00	
10:00 – 12:00	
12:00 – 14:00	
14:00 – 16:00	
16:00 – 18:00	
18:00 – 20:00	
20:00 – 22:00	
22:00 – 00:00	

Future:

00:00 – 02:00	
02:00 – 04:00	
04:00 – 06:00	
06:00 – 08:00	
08:00 – 10:00	
10:00 – 12:00	
12:00 – 14:00	
14:00 – 16:00	
16:00 – 18:00	
18:00 – 20:00	
20:00 – 22:00	
22:00 – 00:00	

The 'Alarm Clock' Theory

You've looked at your relationship with medication. You've considered your supporting therapy options. You've co-opted a pretty useful 'mantra' if I say so myself ("This. Then that."). You've laid down some foundations around your catastrophic thinking and you've looked at goal setting and an alternative approach to time management. You've done *a lot* so far, yeah? All you've got to do now is get up and get going... Sounds easy, right?

How we wake up each day or how we're woken up *matters*. It sounds almost simplistic and arbitrary to say it but so many of us don't seem to lay a lot of importance around this as much as we probably should. How often have we slept in for work or an appointment and had to switch immediately from deep slumber to rushing at 100mph to get showered, fed and out the door for the day with the high-speed stress of it all taking a while to shake off? How often have we woken too soon, watched the bedside clock tick away time that could have been spent sleeping then when you finally drift back off the alarm blares you back awake and you feel half-dazed and thoroughly unrested?

When I was fifteen years old my father broke my nose.

It was the first of four times I'd get my nose broken and I'm still amazed to this day that it looks as physically tolerable in the middle of my face as it does, all things considered.

It was late on a Saturday night.

The local pub had called 'last orders' and I'd had an atypical Saturday night in alone – looking out my bedroom window discreetly from the corner of the blinds so that no tilt could be seen to the outside world, watching the kids from my school congregate on the grass at the edge of the local park to illicitly drink cider, get loud and 'get it on' with each other.

A social gathering that felt so foreign and miles away to me. Yet it was 100 metres or less from my bedroom window. After routinely depressing myself with this act once more and after being sure my parents had left for the evening and my sister was out, I'd venture downstairs and click the TV on.

Because Saturday nights were 'Sky Movies Premiere' night.

If you're an 80s kid who saw out your teens in the early 1990s and your parents had Sky during that time, then you'll definitely have that certain rotation of films from around then that are burnt into your affections due to Sky having a very limited library and playing the same films incessantly for months on end. And Saturday evenings were always the same family film at six, big premiere at eight, mindless action straight-to-video type shite at ten and then a bit of soft porn at midnight.

There are some films from that era that I have great fondness for as a result. See the Joe Pesci comedy The Super, Crackerjack (aka Thomas Ian Griffiths' "Die Hard in a ski resort"), Hider In The House (which now makes Gary Busey look *sane*) and Night of the Running Man (or 'No Country For Old Men before there was a No Country For Old Men' for video junkies of the 1990s) as examples. Others like Midnight Sting, Surviving The Game, Rapid Fire, Judgment Night, Clifford and The Blade have ascended higher and become all-time favourite films of mine.

Ricochet is up there as like the 'grandaddy' of 'em *all*!

Ricochet is Russell Mulcahy's giddy slice of shocking ridiculousness that followed his double-whammy of Razorback and Highlander and the nightmare production on Highlander II.

It is a gloriously unashamed, absolutely bonkers action thriller; a gratuitously violent and excessively ridiculous confection of insanity married to stupidity...

Denzel Washington is at the peak of his sexy-as-fuck, charisma drenched masculinity! John Lithgow delivers yet another of his marvellous psycho turns! The underwear face-off that serves as what a 'normal' film would refer to as the "instigating act"? The heavy lay-up of the Watts Towers in that way that has you thinking [correctly] "That must be where the climax is going to be"? The not-at-all-relevant prison swordfights with armour made of phonebooks and instruction manuals? Denzel getting raped whilst hopped up on an enforced dose of heroin so he can be given a mega splash of gonorrhoea? Ice-T doing a very *special* type of 'acting' that many would describe as “not being able to act” whilst Kevin Pollak sets up his position as 'The Greatest Sidekick of the 1990s'? Mary Ellen Trainor cameoing as Gail Wallens from Die Hard, making this a secret Die Hard sequel and... I could wax lyrical about Ricochet for *a whole book*, but I digress.

On this particular Saturday night, I was poorly and had been left medication by my mum to take alongside some cough medicine. I spilt some of the cough medicine, cleaned it up and unlocked the back door to hide the ‘clean up’ evidence by burying it deep in the bin outside lest I got a smack for having wasted the medicine. I locked the door behind me afterwards – and stupidly left the key in the door.

This would be a mistake that would cost me dearly and leave me psychologically damaged for many years to come.

You see, an hour or so after locking the back door I felt poorly enough that I decided to go to bed.

Normally the routine was that my mum and dad would roll in from the pub just after midnight, point at me on the sofa and bark “Bed!” and I’d obediently and immediately exit the living room and hand the TV off to my dad for him to watch the Match of the Day episode he’d taped whilst he was out. But by the time they returned home, I was in bed asleep.

Zonked out.

And I mean *unconscious* to the war breaking out around me.

My mum and dad were banging on the door, banging on the windows, throwing stones up at my bedroom. They couldn't get their key in to unlock the door because mine was in the lock on the other side. They hadn't taken the keys for the other entrance with them. I didn't hear anything. I was *out*.

The banging apparently woke the neighbours, people started coming out in the street. It was as embarrassing as embarrassing could get for my parents – them being the sort of people who lived to be one step up the rung of respectability and 'class' from those around them.

And now a neighbour is lending my dad a ladder so that he can climb up and get in through a partially open bathroom window, jeered by other people in the street whilst he did this because my dad was no longer a slim man and that is being polite. All the while, I snored away...

... Right up until I was startled awake suddenly by my bedroom door bursting open, smashing off the wall with speed and a massive bang as a figure ran out of the darkness and crunched me right in the centre of my face with a heavy blow.

I remember gasping and trying to recoil with the shock and the fear as this figure grabbed my hair, held me in place and punched me two more times before allowing me to drop back down onto the pillow.

I began to violently shake. I recall that vividly.

Someone had got into the house and attacked me.

They were still in the house. I could hear them.

I pulled the duvet over my head, terrified that they were going to come back to kill me once they'd finished ransacking the house.

Just then my duvet lit up from my bedroom light being switched on. I heard my mother's voice calling me a "stupid shit". I looked out from underneath the duvet and she instantly screamed.

She screamed my dad's name and followed it with "What have you done?"

My dad entered the room with blood on his fist and I saw the colour drain from his face.

It was then I looked down at myself and realised I was drenched in blood. There was blood up the wall next to where I had lain. I gave myself over to the immense pain in the centre of my face and the crippling headache as the shock subsided slightly.

My mother got me up and took me into the bathroom where she showered me down whilst my dad stripped my bed. All the while she barked at my dad, demanding to know how they were going to explain away my face. "You took it too far!" she shouted. "Too far?" my dad bellowed back. "I've nearly broken my neck climbing through that window! He embarrassed us in front of the whole street." "That doesn't mean you get to spread his nose across his face!" she replied.

I caught a look of myself in the mirror.

My nose was three times its size.

I'd come to have my nose broke three more times after this. Once due to being attacked at school, once on a night out gifted to me by the fella my then-girlfriend was cheating on me with and once because of a short-lived boxing career, representing the uniformed services in a tournament. None of them hurt anything like *this*.

I spent the rest of the night sat wide awake, staring at my bedroom door, eventually getting up and putting the light on and moving my desk chair against the door – just to slow down anyone coming through next time. The following morning, I came downstairs swollen and bruised to be told by my mum that I was going to hospital to get my nose checked and that I needed to understand "the story"; how I'd got up in the middle of the night, full of cold, to go downstairs and get a glass of water and that I'd fell down the stairs and hit my face.

At the hospital the attending doctor was astute enough to connect the knuckle marking underneath my eye with the developing bruising on my dad's hand, as he sat in the chair next to me.

He said that it was "NHS Policy" that he had to do a "welfare check" and asked my parents to leave the room momentarily. As soon as they did the doctor asked who had hit me.

I lied by sticking to my mum's version of events. He stared at me and slowly nodded his head. "Your parents didn't do this to you? You've not been in a fight with anyone?"

I shook my head, whilst internally I wanted to point at my dad through the door and scream "HE DID IT!" The doctor forced a smile and said, "Just a fight with the stairs then?" and opened the door for my parents to come back in. I think back often to what would've happened, Sliding Doors style, if I had spoken up for myself there and then in that moment. Would my parents have been prosecuted? Would I have been taken away from them? Would I have been allowed to go and live with my grandparents?

The following week I was woken in the night from the sound of our bin falling over in the wind beneath my bedroom window. I sat bolt upright in bed and saw that I was urinating myself with fear. The resounding mockery and fury from my parents and my sister the next morning showed they were oblivious or unwilling to make any sort of connection between the events of the preceding weekend and this incident.

My father's attack on me destroyed my ability to sleep deeply for over two decades. I took to sleeping with a pillow underneath the door to semi-block it from opening properly. I got used to surviving on four to five hours of sleep from lying in bed, staring at the entrance / exit point of wherever I was staying, until I eventually passed out from exhaustion.

By the point you could add the 'night terrors' resultant from my experiences in the military and uniformed services, I was a barely functioning insomniac by the age of twenty-five.

Still to this day, although better than I was, if I'm woken too suddenly or abrasively (certainly by someone touching me or shaking me – which is really *something* once you've had kids, let me tell you!) my entire body is prone to bracing at the same time I gasp so quickly I can be left having to steady my breath for minutes afterwards.

It taints the start of a day and can affect my mindset emotionally quite considerably.

So, trust me when I say I take the 'wake up' experience, the quality of it and the 'science' behind it very seriously indeed. For highly personal reasons if nothing else.

I learnt that in some Japanese cultures alarms are poorly thought of. It's especially considered offensive and ill-mannered amongst the Japanese to have a meeting or social engagement interrupted by abradant and harsh alarm chimes or notification sounds.

The National Institute of Industrial Health in Japan did a study that showed daily use of alarms had a negative impact on our lives and that being awoken *suddenly* or from a deep state of sleep was dangerous to our health. Which shouldn't come as a surprise really, should it? The sudden audible jolt brings a waking start to our day with a rushed increase of our heart rate and our blood pressure. The adrenaline puts us in a starting position of stress.

None of these things will do well to your long term health anyway (more so because as our blood thickens from lying still during the night a ballistically speeded increase in pressure / rate cannot be good), but if you're someone who's suffering from poor mental health and its brought about insomnia or poor sleep hygiene that's only going to multiply problems; imagine spending hours trying to get to sleep but routinely getting stuck ruminating and worrying then eventually dozing off in the early hours and after three hours you're blasted awake by a rock song or the jazziest and loudest notification option built into your phone to minimise your chance of sleeping through.

That was *my* biggest problem – an inability to get to sleep and then when I would eventually go under almost by way of exhaustive 'collapse' rather than choice, the sleep wouldn't be restorative, and I would be startled awake by an alarm that shook me so suddenly into consciousness my immediate starting thought was that my father was in the room attacking me again.

This continued into my thirties before I got control of it.

The more I started reading up on the Japanese 'take' on sleep, wakening and alarms the more I started to think about the way we structure how we wake from an emotional and mental perspective.

The Japanese promote the notion of waking to nature sounds and natural light, and by making the right choices in your life to know what your 'reason for being' (ikigai) is so you come to wake naturally and enthusiastically, *wanting* to start your day.

I'll not try to drag you so far over to that line of thought. But what I will say is there is *something* to finding 'that' song that fits the criteria of having a subtle aural quality or musical build to it yet also you have a positive emotional attachment to. By choosing to start the day with that song – and finding that 'one' is part of the fun and a journey through the memory banks in itself – you're easing into consciousness on a happy memory, which is no bad way to start the day is it? Hey, it's certainly better than a broken nose.

What about the song that you had your first kiss to? (Mine was Boy Meets Girl's 'Waiting For A Star To Fall') Or the song you had your first dance to on your wedding day? The song you remember from a really good holiday?

Your 'alarm' song choice should be personal to *you*. Are you seeing the pattern yet on this mental health journey – like your goals and your challenges, it is *all* personal to you. To each their absolute own. Whatever the reason, it just needs to cue you out of your slumber in a non-abrasive way and with *some* thought to the person next to you in bed.

For a while I used to start my day with Hans Zimmer's 'Show Me Your Firetruck' from the 1991 film Backdraft.

Backdraft has a tremendous studio blockbuster that holds up to this day and has a terrific musical score.

Its magnificence in that regard is reflected in the fact it was repurposed for nearly every movie trailer for the whole of the 1990s, until Crimson Tide's score came along... also by Hans Zimmer!

But I digress. Again.

You're beginning to see why some of my friends now refer to me as 'Ronnie Corbett', right? And if you can't it's because you're too young to get the reference and you should stop making the rest of us feel so goddamn old.

I chose 'Show Me Your Firetruck' because of the slow, quiet build into something adrenalised once I'd stirred and got me going for the day.

Then I moved in with my now wife and within a couple of months she told me that my alarm was, quote unquote, "making [her] not like Backdraft and that was unforgiveable because Backdraft is great."

I have one friend who upon learning of my alarm clock 'theory' set about using The Beatles' 1967 song 'Getting Better' from Sgt Pepper's Lonely Hearts Club Band (sample lyrics: "I've got to admit it's getting better. A little better all the time, it can't get no worse. I have to admit it's getting better. It's getting better...") and now swears that his mornings are much improved because of this. I guess you could say his mornings "got better"? Go figure.

I tried using 'Peace of Mind' by Boston, from their 1976 self-titled album, because I attempted to will myself into believing that the lyrics were super-relevant to my life as it was at the time and how I was feeling.

(Sample lyrics: "Now if you're feelin' kinda low 'bout the dues you've been paying. Future's coming much too slow, and you wanna run, but somehow you just keep on stayin'. Can't decide on which way to go. Yeah, yeah, yeah...")

Which is a terrible thing to do because you think shit like that helps but in reality, it's just reinforcing a negative feeling.

Also, that hard intro on 'Peace of Mind' could cause you to turn the bedsheets brown in shock if you're in a deep enough sleep. Trust me, I've come close. Too many times.

The song that got me considering the notion of your morning 'theme song', so to speak, was 'Real Gone Kid' by Deacon Blue from their 1989 album When The World Knows Your Name.

It was my morning alarm for the longest time and even at the point it was driving my wife bonkers I couldn't give up on being roused awake by it. (I'd sacrificed Hans Zimmer's 'Show Me Your Firetruck' to her grumbles, this felt a step too far.)

I realised that it was because it took me back to being on the boxing team during my military days, and training with the same 'mixtape' playing every day with the same tracks on it...

'Get Up' by Mike & The Mechanics, 'Don't Stop Believing' by Journey, 'Grand Illusion' by Styx and 'Real Gone Kid' by Deacon Blue stand out. This was not a compilation that had been made by a young person, but unlike others on the team I loved it.

This song reminded me of a big achievement I'd made. It's slow build in eased me awake without any shock or trauma. It put me in a good mood.

That was the song that made me think about the 'science' around how we stir from sleep and how we start our day.

Since I developed this theory around the sounds we start our day with, my alarm nowadays is Terry Bush's theme song from the revival of The Littlest Hobo. (I say revival because I only learnt recently that the 1979 – 1985 version was actually a 'redo' of a show that originally ran from 1963 to 1965. Did *you* know that?).

The alarm goes off and I hear "There's a voice, that keeps on calling me. Down the road, that's where I'll always be. Every stop I make, I make a new friend. Can't stay for long, just turn around and I'm gone again." and I'm immediately reminded of sitting cuddled with my grandma on the sofa as a child, feeling *safe*.

It's a good memory and a great trigger to accessing it. And that's exactly in theory what your least abrasive 'alarm' song should be.

I say that your choice should be entirely personal to you but remember to spare a thought as to who you're waking up next to. And in some ways what your emotional relationship is to the song, I guess.

In my early thirties, I dated a woman who had *a lot* of problems going on in her life. And think about this – if **I'm** saying you've got a lot of problems then you know something is fucked up!

The one I could not seem to move past was that she was really into the song 'The Climb' by Miley Cyrus. The 2009 'MTV Movie Award for Best Song From a Movie' / 'Teen Choice Award for Best Single' winner, taken from the major motion picture Hannah Montana: The Movie. And I mean like… *really* into it too.

It was the alarm on her phone, sure. But it was also central to her personal teachings. And that was a *bit* weird to me.

Which is obviously very hypocritical coming from someone who's written an entire book around the principles that Die Hard can fundamentally be used as a supportive tool for drawing improvement in your mental health. I know. I accept that. I think I could've coped with starting each day with 'The Climb' by Miley Cyrus because, if we're honest, Miley Cyrus' 'The Climb' is a frickin' *great* song, man.

But this woman made it all weird.

She talked about 'The Climb' by Miley Cyrus all the time.

All. The. Time.

It just seemed to work its way into every conversation or get played in the car whenever we were going somewhere.

One time I had come in from a really bad day at work and I was stressed out because I was covering two other members of staff's workload whilst they were off sick and bosses were setting unrealistic targets and I just wanted to come in, crack a beer and have a bit of a 'moan' to depressurise from the day before starting it all over again tomorrow.

After whining a little bit, my then girlfriend replied with *two-thousand percent earnestness* "It sounds like it's always going to be an uphill battle and sometimes you're going to have to lose."

And just as my eyebrows arched and I exhaled my cigarette she continued "But it isn't how fast you get there, it's about what's waiting on the other side."

I slowly nodded, tried to bite down on my lip but instead simply asked "Did you just quote 'The Climb' by Miley Cyrus to me?" She replied, "Maybe not consciously?"

We broke up a couple of weeks later. I told her it was because of trust issues due to how she repeatedly tried and sometimes succeeded in kissing all and sundry when she'd had so much as two drinks.

But really, all these years later, I think I'm willing to admit it was definitely because of the whole obsession with 'The Climb' by Miley Cyrus.

"I Feel Seen" #3

THE BEST OF TIMES

My grandfather got me into boxing as a teenager. I was getting mercilessly bullied at school and as an ex-military PT and navy boxer himself he was slowly getting pissed off at my inability / unwillingness to defend myself.

It started with him showing me how to throw a punch and his excitement at discovering I was a southpaw took us from there, basically.

I enjoyed learning combinations from my grandad, I liked becoming educated to the 'sweet science' of it all and, I'm not going to lie, I really leaned in to how things improved at school when I followed my grandad's advice of putting the biggest one in the group of bullies down with a punch in the school yard and watching the cowardice of the others cause them to scatter and leave me alone thereafter.

My dad nearly ruined it for me. He was never one for letting me take part in a sport for the *enjoyment* of it.

Everything had to be competitive. Whatever I did had to be measured against the standards of other people's kids:

I did well on school sports' day at the hurdles, next thing you know he was taking me up to the athletics track and running timed drills. I made the reserve roster for the school cricket team; he went out and bought me a bat and made me practise stances and swings in the living room for nearly an hour every night.

He would go from showing me no interest whatsoever other than when it was time to smack me around for some infraction I'd committed...

... to suddenly *obsessively* coaching me on whatever sport I'd so much as looked in the direction of.

At first, I embraced his efforts because I wanted a 'connection' with my father so badly that my feeling was I would take it any way I could get it. But it quickly became oppressive and would swiftly descend into me being dragged around by the scruff of my neck whilst he barked "Again. Do it again. But do it right."

I loved goalkeeping in football, and I was good at in the eyes of my school PE teacher. Not in the eyes of my father though and his endless re-training of my abilities eventually killed any interest I had in it.

With boxing simply training in it with my grandfather for the purposes of self-defence and enjoyment wasn't enough for my dad and soon he was driving me around the handful of boxing clubs in the region, trying to find one that would take me on and develop me. I didn't know that I wanted to box competitively.

I was fourteen years of age and suddenly, I was being pushed swiftly from shadowboxing in my grandad's living room to sparring with other kids, and frequently getting my arse handed to me.

I got good though.

Well, I got *reasonably* good.

I won some fights. I lost some fights. I had developed a style of boxing that meant I had no long-term viability in the ring – I would absorb a heavy plethora of blows early on and have an innate ability to pull back from the beating and, at the exact moment an opponent's arms would slow from rapid exertion, fit in tight and sharp combinations that served me well.

You couldn't box like that with continuing regularity though.

The body and the brain can't sustain that.

I used my upcoming GCSEs as an 'out' from continuing to box at competition level, much to my dad's fury.

I never gave boxing another thought until I joined the military three years later.

As was the standard for me, I struggled to make friends upon joining and I really struggled to fit in within the military structure.

Within the first couple of weeks of 'boot camp' (or basic training) my Sergeant claimed there was a "Mahoney from Police Academy type in every cohort and [I] was [his]".

He vowed to break me quickly and make me scared to speak without thinking of him first, which he did with ease through additional locker inspections that trashed / smashed my carefully bulled and ironed kit as well as 'hose downs' with cold water whilst the rest of my fellow recruits stood on parade watching.

I didn't know who to be or how to act. I just knew instantly that I was in the *wrong* environment, but I was too scared to leave for fear of having to face my parents' disappointment.

I retreated inwards and routinely ate at the edge of the huge, long tables away from everyone else and would sneak off base under the guise of going for a run but really take a bus into the small town centre to watch a film in their tiny cinema on my own.

I was neither a good nor natural solider and would often only pass my assessments after I'd got verbally ripped to shreds on the re-sit by my instructors, who'd come to nickname me 'Honey Monster' after the mascot from the Sugar Puffs breakfast cereal - because I was apparently "a big, bumbling lunk that crashed [my] way through everything".

I became so desperate for some form of connection after a while that when I saw the notice that the boxing team were holding trials, I decided to give it a try as a means of making friends.

Think about that – I was going to voluntarily get punched in the face to win friends and influence people! I made the reserve team and started to train regularly. Doing so made not one jot in terms of my connections with anyone though it got me in the best shape I've ever been in even to this day.

Only the regular 'A-team' boxers got to train "full time" and be let free from their trade.

The rest of us had to fit in circuit training and the like in our lunch-hours or after shift in our down time.

Six weeks out from an upcoming tri-military competition one of the 'A-team' boxers got injured and I was pulled up from the reserves to take his slot.

Boxing at a weight outside of what I was used to and against an opponent who was *infamous* – he had never been beaten by anybody, had never been knocked down and no one had ever got past the second round with him! In the eyes of the coaches that suddenly and reluctantly had to take me on I was just to "hold and endure as best [I] could" for the sake of overall 'points', save forfeiting.

In *my* eyes, this was my Rocky moment... stacked odds, wildcard shot, low expectations, formidable opponent... I was *so* deluded that my delusion proved infectious and before I know it one Warrant Officer running the team had taken me under his wing properly and decided we were going to "go for it" (Rocky quote intentional).

I can see your eyes are starting to glaze over a bit and you're starting to get restless as to where the connection is to Ron Shelton's 1986 almost forgotten sports comedy so I'll just jump to the 'third act':

I fought this guy with everything I had. He was three inches taller than me, wider than me and his arms seemed to go on forever. The first punch he threw actually cracked my right eye socket.

Seriously.

I knew in that moment that I was dangerously, *dangerously* out of my depth and my search for human connection, validation, greatness or whatever you want to dress it up as had taken me too far into a direction that could possibly get me killed.

The atmosphere was charged too.

The crowd was mostly my opponent's service colleagues more than mine and mine weren't exactly audibly in my corner anyway.

I was getting jeered and booed whilst getting lathered with punches at a speed and force I'd never been hit with in my life, and my dad was no lightweight I assure you.

I knew I couldn't do my old tactic of 'soaking it up and striking late' so I started fighting back as best I could, as well as I could muster... and it started to seem like what I could muster was good enough.

My corner team barked these random non-sequiturs ("Everything for now!" "Leave nothing behind!" "Hold your line!") that still echo in my head to this day, don't really make a whole heap of sense in or out of context but adrenalised me back then in a very weird way.

Before I knew it, I was passed the point anyone had ever got with this guy. I'd hung in longer than any other opponent he fought, and I was still conscious.

I decided regardless of anything else I was going to go all the way with him. Not sexually. I mean all the way to the final bell. I don't know why I didn't just say that in the first place. Or why I felt I had to clarify it. As if the length of this anecdote wasn't enough of a problem, now I've made it awkward too. Sorry. Anyway...

The crowd turned ever so slightly in my favour. My corner team were going crazy at the prospect of this turning into an upset no one could have predicted. The other guy was starting to slacken by letting his frustrations get to him and then... BOOM! ... He went down and the whole place lit up with screams, cheers, jeers, you name it.

Now, let me be clear here, he got up on the count of four, went on to win on points and maintains to this day that he *slipped* and was not knocked down but I know what I know – I can still feel the impact of my left hand hitting the side of his head, right in the sweet spot between his jaw and his forehead and my right swiftly following with an uppercut straight to the centre of his jaw like the combination was designed by the Gods themselves... and he went down.

No one had gone past the second round with this guy. *I* had.

No one had ever knocked him down. *I* had.

For all of five seconds I genuinely thought I was going to win this thing, but he responded to the embarrassment of what had happened to him with a flurry that left me with a broken rib, a broken nose and a damaged rotator cuff, amongst other things that later needed stitched and iced.

The fight ended and my name was being cheered despite having lost. I returned to the changing room and was treated like a hero by the other members of the boxing team.

The other coaches were complimenting me and ruffling my hair, helping me attach ice packs and get in a comfortable position. For the next couple of weeks, I was treated as if I was a *golden god* on the military base, I couldn't pay for a drink or walk anyway. It was all free pints and lifts to wherever I was going. It was less than 10 minutes of my life that had added up to 166,554 hours and 999,3240 minutes at that point yet back then they were the greatest 10 minutes I had ever lived. All of the pain, the changed gait, the slight permanent disfiguring of my face... it was all worth it just to have been lauded like that and to now be looked at in this way.

And just as soon as it all finally arrived for me, it went away.

People moved on. Other things happened. Other sporting achievements within the service occurred. Its significance was only significant to me, and, within a couple of months, my career was done, and my mental health kicked off the rails anyway. It just... disappeared from everywhere but my memory. Pretty soon I was just this depressive, barely employed drunk back up in my hometown who'd get soused then regale the same friends with the same 'My Rocky Moment' yarn.

I had a video tape of the fight. I showed it to my friends when I first returned home. In fact, I showed it to them so often that they genuinely started to brace against my suggestion to watch it for the thirteenth, fourteenth or fifteenth time.

I would often sit alone drunk, watching it and rewinding certain bits. I was so out of shape and far gone in my depression at this point that I didn't recognise the person in the video anymore.

I would fixate on the very moment on the tape that captured the moment when I stood up for the final round and you could visibly see me pull myself up, straighten up through the pain and the broken rib and the ripped out shoulder.

At the exact moment that the 'me' in the video would start stepping forward out of his corner I would burst into tears and drunkenly mutter "What was in *that* guy? Where's *that* gone? Why don't I have *that* anymore?"

I eventually broke the tape.

Ron Shelton writes and sometimes directs these great movies about men and their feelings, and their hopes and aspirations. And he dresses them up in the disguise of a sports movie.

Everyone will tell you that his masterpiece in this regard is Bull Durham but that's not true. It is *really* Tin Cup, a beautiful sporting underdog film with a heart-warming romance at the centre of it – using golfing as metaphors for life and love.

In the mid-80s he wrote a by-the-numbers sports comedy with a great hook and handed it off to Roger Spottiswoode to direct, about a middle-aged banker called Jack Dundee (Robin Williams) who lives in a small rust-belt American town where football is 'everything' and for which he's still regarded year after year as the town 'joke' because he dropped an important pass during the biggest high school football game and cost the town a championship. They've never let him forget it, he's never been able to get over it and now in his forties he decides that he's going to recruit the old high school quarterback and local legend Reno Hightower (Kurt Russell) to stage a rematch of the game with the same now-aged players so he can have a shot at redemption.

Like with Tin Cup, Ron Shelton's written a script that you 'age' into rather than appreciate outright. Beneath the surface though lies something more.

I loved this movie as a kid because I was then and remain now a Robin Williams obsessive but as an adult I came to love it more.

The notion of hitting adulthood with nothing but a lifetime of regret, your biggest mistake(s) sitting on your chest like the weight of two trucks and a crippling depression born from having to live as a total joke to those around you? Wow! This was about *me*!

Hidden away inside the film there's a lovely underlining moral about facing down those regrets.

Reno Hightower:
"I was never great. I was pretty good. I was great for around here. Every year I got better. The people remember me in my prime. The kids always ask me about the 6 touchdown passes against Porterville. Hell, I only threw 3 touchdowns."

Jack Dundee:
"It was 7."

Reno Hightower:
"I'm not going to argue. I like the idea of 7 better. In a couple more years it'll be 8. I get better with age. My knees are killing me. I'm slow."

Jack Dundee:
"That's why you didn't want to play the game."

Reno Hightower:
"No. I just... I didn't want to destroy the only thing I've got left - those stories about how great I was."

Within a *terrific* cast (Holly Palance, Donald Moffatt, the late great Margaret Whitton, M. Emmet Walsh, Donovan Scott, Kirk Cameron and Robyn Lively) Pamela Reed stands out to remind you she was one of the great unsung talents of the 80s / 90s... That made it sound like Pamela Reed is dead. Far from it. She's *really* tremendous here and steals scenes left right and centre, which is very impressive when she's sharing those scenes with Kurt Russell and Robin Williams.

Williams' performance touches base with all the silliness audiences wanted from him back then, but with a huge dollop of heart too. The Best of Times is *quintessential* Kurt Russell though. He's so good at what he does by making it all look so effortless, and that's on show here.

I watched The Best of Times again as an adult and I saw so much of myself in Williams' Jack Dundee:

How he was treated by the townsfolk was how I was treated by family, how he regarded himself was how I considered myself and the weight of what he carried upon himself to the point it was obsessional and off-putting to people was something that was very familiar to me.

Which is why I got up out of bed one morning and decided I too was going to have my moment back – I was going to return to boxing!

All the barriers that would have stopped a more sensible person didn't deter me one bit.

Who cares that I was smoking a pack and a half of Lucky Strike Lights a day? Or drinking four cans of Heineken (minimum), not counting Jim Beam, per night? Or eating out of a takeaway box or a Doritos bag for nearly every meal – if I was eating at all? And hadn't exercised in about six years or so at that point.

I didn't go and join a boxing club and start training again either. No, of course I didn't. I went barrelling around the internet whilst three sheets to the wind on lager and bourbon one night and found some unlicensed events being held. There were some that skirted damn close to ostensibly being organised bare-knuckle brawls. There were some that were a little bit higher up the chain than that. I found a 'classy' looking one that gave out trophies and all sorts. And I registered for it – with ten days to train.

For about a week I would try to go for runs and I would shadow box in my flat alone. I tried to tighten up my diet a little bit. It all went about as well as training montages go for a guy who had cut down to smoking just a pack of Lucky Strike Lights and had given up the Heineken (but kept up the Jim Beam to help put me to sleep). And then ten days later I drove fifty to sixty miles down south on my own... and *boxed.*

I vomited my way through the rounds.

And miraculously got myself out of there with far less injuries all things considered, solely because the people I fought were less experienced than me and a tiny bit easier to control.

I came away with a couple of trophies (no, I've no idea how either) as well as this 'buzz' that carried me back home afterwards.

But it didn't fulfil me the way I wanted it to. The answers or solutions didn't lie with me getting 'knocked around' and it didn't set me back down a boxing path or provide me any redemption like it did for Jack Dundee. I came home that night, I poured myself a larger Jim Beam than normal and flopped down in front of the TV. And within a couple of hours, despite boxing trophies sat on the coffee table in front of me, I was back to thinking about what a 'loser' I was and how 'pathetic' I was.

Decades later and I watch The Best of Times now with a feeling of pride in a lot of ways. I don't look back under a filter of 'failure'. I look back and think about the guy who was that depressed, that far down a bottle and that out of shape and one day he still simply got up, went out and *fought*.

Literally.

I look back on that guy, remind myself that the guy was me and that it took some resolve and courage (and, okay, a heady dash of stupidity too) to do that.

And I cut myself a little slack.

Sometimes I do this by pretending that out there on some military base tucked away on the outskirts of some nondescript British village is an old sweat of a serviceman who's put most of his time in, rose to a respectful enough rank and is now waiting out his last couple of years before retirement doing 'corner-work' on a military boxing team, and every now and again he pulls out the "old stories" for a couple of the up-and-comers, wannabes or contenders. And maybe... just... maybe... on one of those occasions he tells the story of ol' Leonard McClane coming out of nowhere to tear the roof of the place going toe-to-toe with the best there was.

And there and then in those moments of kidding myself, I realise I always thought I was Jack Dundee but I'm actually more like Reno Hightower, because just like him the "stories" can often mean something important to us regardless of how much time gets in the way.

The Cost of a Text

Most people nowadays don't pay for a text, do they? They come as some unlimited deal on your phone. And then there's WhatsApp, which has predominantly replaced the old text messaging thing and... and... Look, what I'm saying is I *acknowledge* that this chapter heading needs work, okay? I get it. The sentiment behind it stands though.

What's the sentiment?

Well, *maybe* we'd be on to discussing that by now if you'd not made me self-conscious about the whole "Texts don't cost!" / "No one texts anymore, *Grandad*!" chapter heading.

I digress.

I don't have many friends but the ones I do have I hold tightly and care for dearly because no matter how far I've progressed in terms of my self-esteem, there is *still* a little part of me that remains so pleased they've chosen to be friends with me at all. I'm certainly not anyone's 'ideal' design of the perfect friend, by any stretch.

One of my longest 'serving' / standing friends is a bloke I've known since I was 14 years of age. We weren't *close* friends growing up. We were hardened movie geeks from a young age who could smell 'our own' within the vicinity of the school corridors and we sniffed each other out, recognising in the other that here was the type of person you could go up to and say "The service number on the bus is 25 25 in the movie Speed, which adds up to 50. And that's the exact miles per hour the bus can't drop below without exploding!" and they'd reply "Woah." And not "Alright, calm down Rain Man!"

We grew older with each other 'just over there' on the side lines of our respective lives, a standing 'date' every three to six months of getting together for a couple of beers and a screening of a movie that no one else would hold any interest in seeing with either of us.

(Like the night we headed out with excitement at the prospect of catching a rare screening of the 1961 Johnny Cash crime movie, Five Minutes To Live, at a fleapit arthouse just outside the city. Or the time we travelled to Glasgow to watch Joe Dante's The Movie Orgy, an infamous nigh-on *seven hour* montage of vintage commercials and TV show clips married with scenes from 1950s b-movies to create a unique collage of visuals about aliens / monsters destroying America.)

He is a dear friend and someone I care about deeply, but we initially (and by initially I mean "the first twenty-five years") never had 'that' sort of friendship where we talked about feelings and troubles, etc.

We dropped in and out of each other's lives and talked about Martin Scorsese and John Carpenter when we saw each other, but at the worst of my mental health issues he was not someone I would burden or go to.

There was a latent part of me that always felt I *shouldn't* because I cherished the friendship we had so much and for so long that I never wanted to risk losing that by presenting myself as wallowing in his company and driving him away finally like I had done with so many other people over the years.

Then one day I was due to meet up with him for one of our bi-annual movie and beer get-togethers and I had to cancel because my mental health was particularly bad. I hadn't left the house in a while, and I knew my depression was quite severe because I was struggling to connect with and concentrate on films. He texted me to confirm arrangements and caught me at one of my more vulnerable moments, I cancelled on him and for the first time ever in our friendship I explained why and that I was grappling with my mental health.

He replied back: "We don't have to do a film. We can just sit and talk if you feel up to it?"

I thanked him and said I'd think about it, later accepting that I had missed him and catching up with him was something I had been looking forward to before I had fell into this depression. I pushed myself to go just for a couple of beers and my friend pulled me back from a dangerous brink that night without intrusive questions, judgement or any sort of dominant push with advice - and probably without even realising he did save me in a lot of ways, because he's humble like that!

He simply listened.

This friend's 'superpower' even to this day lies simply in taking the time to be present in my life and to hold conversations about a multitude of different things around our shared interests as well as mental health. Occasionally, at the worst of my catastrophising and harshest of verbal self-flagellations, he would quietly present an alternative line of thought or a suggestion that was just gently put out there before me to take or leave.

And because when our mental health is at its worse we are prone to always look to the negative, I can assure you that I came away from those beers bemoaning the fact that I had access to such a wonderful source of support for these last thirty or so years and I'd never realised it was there or been open and transparent enough with the person in question to access it before.

One of the biggest lines of bullshit that exists around mental health when it comes to feeling depressed, lonely, stressed, anxious and the like is that "misery loves company". It *really* doesn't. It absolutely does not. Company helps lessen the weight of an emotional load and misery does not want that to happen because the lighter the load on your mental health the sparser the breeding ground it can exist within.

Misery doesn't love company.

Misery loves loneliness and darkness.

Misery loves the blinds shut and the curtains drawn so you can't catch sight of something in the 'outside world' that triggers a pleasant memory or a feeling of hope, the quietness of an empty room to make you feel lonelier than you actually are, a barrage of self-defining negative thoughts that go uninterrupted so you don't have an opportunity to challenge or fact-check them... *that's* what misery loves.

So, misery definitely doesn't want you to reach out to other people.

It thrives on making you believe that you don't in fact *have* other people which, separate to the damage it used to do to my self-esteem, was one of the most successful ways of getting to me at my lowest points.

Which is what makes that one single text to someone saying "Hey, I'm not having a good time at the moment and could do with talking to someone. Can I buy you a coffee?" such an important (and courageous!) thing to do.

Anything mental health related can be disconcerting to some people and their response to seeing someone struggle is one that looks to the common eye like they're looking in the other direction.

The likelihood however is that they're uncomfortable because they're worried; they don't know what to say and there's a legitimate fear in some people that they might say the wrong thing or give the wrong advice and it may result in a depressed person harming themselves.

They're frightened, so they pull away. Unlike my family who routinely did not want to help because they found it "embarrassing".

This is why it is important that you are considered in who you approach within your group of friends.

The contact should be with someone you trust and someone you value because the support they provide has got to be something that you embrace or are willing to try to.

There is going to be a vastly better outcome from you reaching out to the friend you've known for some time and have a measure of their personality and perspective over the work colleague you only speak to at the photocopier.

Friendship is incredibly important and impactive to those having a low period in their mental health.

We talked earlier about those friendships or influences that may need exorcised because they are damaging your emotional well-being but pulling away, dismantling, or 'killing' an otherwise *fruitful* and *meaningful* friendship can worsen your negative feeling if you're not careful.

I have been prone to feelings of being unworthy of friendship and not having value and it took a long time for me to realise that this was a carry-over from a lot of remarks from my parents growing up around "Who would want to be friends with you when..." or "No wonder no one wants to be your friend when..."

The feeling of unworthiness is a strong barrier to breach, especially when you add on top of it the very common fear of not wanting to burden people with your 'troubles'. Or even that you have no one to burden anyway. These feelings often cause us to push away friends, purposefully or sometimes accidentally, that are trying to help.

We must be careful in doing so at our lowest or most difficult points emotionally because the benefits of friendship on our mental health are difficult to argue against.

A positive friendship can make changes to our brain functions by altering even ever so slightly our thinking habits – the way we have perceived a situation, clarity around a particular feeling and small measures of actualised support in overcoming something that is causing us immense stress.

In the same way that I'll encourage you later on in this book to invest emotionally in films that make you feel empathetic towards the characters or 'seen' in a portrayal on screen, it's important to recognise that there is extreme power in receiving empathy and support from someone in our actual life that we regard or respect also.

You should be willing – as part of your own self-reflection – to challenge your beliefs around what constitutes a friend and a friendship of value.

For example, if you know that alcohol is impacting you badly in your daily life and proving to be a real weapon against you in your battle to take control of your mental health, having that friend who only wants to go out and get 'smashed', "drink away the problems" and can't be negotiated with around this... that friendship probably needs looked at and a few hard questions asked.

The same applies to what and how you *define* a friend. We sometimes seem to have a definition of this formed on what we see on TV or in films, like it must be someone we grew up with, work with or spend a set number of hours with per week / month / year for us to have the sort of bond where trust, respect, affection and the like can be formed. I'm one of those dudes' whose best friend is his wife. If you think she's standing next to me dictating that then you would be *wrong* (... come back in five minutes, she's still standing here!). I'm also someone who considers my father-in-law to be a monumentally important friend in my life because of the advice he provides, the selflessness he displays towards others and his outlook on life that is infectious, inspiring and rewarding.

A friend isn't someone that's defined by anyone else but *you* and your regard for the person. They can be family. Hell, it kills me to say it being a technological caveman in so many ways, but they can even be virtual / online. I have very close friendships with people on the other side of the world that I've never met but who I've 'known' through shared interests across the internet for so many years that a bond has formed and now, we're like weirdo pen-pals who occasionally shift our conversations from talking about a new film we both hated to giving each other advice around raising our children or work-related troubles.

The important thing lies in the trust and esteem you have for a friend.

Because with the click of that 'send' button they're going to be the person that steps up alongside you to look that ol' black cloud of depression in the face and say "Nope, they're *not* alone!" or "See! They *do* have friends!" and even "Look, this one time they helped me move house and now I'm one down to them so I'm here, okay? I'm *here* having to deal with *you*, Misery. So, let's get this over and fucking done with so I can get back to talking about 1980s creature features in the corner of the bar with this guy, alright?"

Set yourself the SMART goal of reaching out to one friend within the next 72 hours. Copy out the 'line', press send, sit back, tick off the SMART goal as complete and feel damn proud of yourself:

> "Hey, I'm not having a good time at the moment and could do with talking to someone. Can I buy you a coffee?"

The Training Montage: Exercise and You

It's a given that exercise is good for you, right? We all *know* that.

But knowing it doesn't make it any easier to *do* when you're naturally inclined to not want to do it or you have a mental health issue that is doing everything in its power to pull you back from doing any – usually with the sort of negative pile-on that used to hobble me all the time:

'What's the point? You're going to do it and you'll just hurt afterwards and it'll not have any positive impact on you anyway because you'll not stick at it and you'll just end up being inconsistent with that like you are everything else! You need to get to a gym if you make any sort of dent on your fitness and you can't afford that right now and... blah, blah, etc. etc'.

Your depression doesn't want you exercising in the same way that household germs don't want you going out to buy cleaning products.

Because the inarguable fact is that it is now wholly proven there is a direct connection between exercise and improved mental health.

Now, come back. Please.

I know how hard some of you will be bracing against what you think is coming next because I've been where you are and if you're reading this then it's likely because you've had some serious problems with your mental health, you feel like you've tried everything else and you're so desperate now you're reading a book by some dude who's claiming Die Hard can help or something...

... and now you're worried because you think I've just waited until 150+ pages into this thing to condescend to you with some version of "Join a gym and tighten up your diet!"

I assure you that's not what this is – unless that's the direction in which you take the advice in this particular chapter.

What I want to be clear about though is exercise as we discuss it going forward doesn't have to hurt, it doesn't have to be huge, it doesn't have to be excessive or expensive. It just needs to be movement, that's it.

Well, movement in line with some modicum of sensible eating. But that's it – *movement*.

You're hearing from someone here who doesn't even *like* exercise. I just have come to understand its intrinsic value in maintaining control over my mental health which is ostensibly what this is all about.

Yeah, I used to box at some minor competitive levels but you're also talking about someone who temporarily set the record in my military boxing team for the fastest road run ever completed... until it was exposed that I had taken a taxi for two-thirds of the route. Because I *hate* running that much and try to actively avoid doing it unless I am being chased.

I am not naturally athletic – as my father would rejoice in telling you, no doubt – and I have no appetite for exercising just for the 'buzz' that comes from 'feeling the burn' or whatever.

I have taken years and years to find a way to exercise for the 'sake' of exercising because I have only ever done so when I had something to train for, a boxing match or a bicycle race or something. I don't have any of those things in my life anymore and I struggled to motivate myself into exercising the minute such things departed.

Once I got a handle over my mental health and the role exercise played in it, I started to realise that I am technically still 'training' for something when I work-out – I'm training to stay alive by having the stamina to stay one step ahead of the mental health issues that I know could kill me if I let them.

There's a *whole heap* of stuff that can and should be said around diet, its relationship to exercise and its effect on our mental health.

The reality however is that I know from personal experience how incredibly difficult it is when trying to find the 'balance' on this journey to incorporate healthy eating and what not.

I'm not a dietician and you're not an idiot. You don't need to be lectured on the inarguable fact that you can't out-train a bad diet, sugary food will crash your mood, eating more than you burn will cause rapid weight gain. You're probably sat right now thinking "This guy wants me to be doing this, that, the other, SMART goals, watch films, go out and see friends and what not... *AND* start cooking healthy, nutritious meals whilst dieting? What the *hell*?"

The truth is no, I just want you to keep it in the back of your mind so that the good work you do in terms of increasing movement, fresh air, trying consistent exercise etc. isn't undone with repeatedly shitty food choices that are doing no good for your mental well-being.

Calorie tracking? Nutrient management? Meal planning and prepping? They're great things to build SMART goals around but remember we're starting small and building upwards so if cooking with consideration and exercise haven't been a part of your life already and you're just starting out they are something you can work towards but just having an *awareness* for now is good enough.

What I want to try and get across to you is that the exercise doesn't have to be classes in a gym when you're feeling self-conscious about yourself or sessions with physical trainers or boot camps that you can't afford. They simply must be more than what you've been doing, which if that was *nothing* then... I think you're going to be okay. That's the mantra we're going to work with going forward:

Always do more than what you did before.

As in always build off from what you last managed.

The professionals call it 'progressive overloading' but we're not going to complicate this.

We're going to keep it *really* basic because:

1. "*motion is lotion, baby*" and

2. modifications when it comes to exercise can have significant supportive impactors on our mental health in a plethora of ways.

The importance of exercise is now more appreciated and valued as a means of treatment within the mental health professional community than it has ever been, and some psychiatrists and doctors believe it has been neglected as a legitimate means of interventive care for too long.

Studies have shown that all forms of exercise are impactive. For a while it was believed the exercise needed to be in excess of twenty minutes daily and of a cardio or aerobic specific nature, but it is now recognised that weight-resistance exercise or simply doing some form of bodyweight driven exercise is just as valuable as swimming, cycling, jogging, etc for reducing anxiety and depression.

Activities such as walking or gardening are equally viable and valuable, especially applied from a starting point of 'nothing at all previously'.

Now the "*science part*" – the mood and emotional improvements are caused by exercise increasing blood circulation to several regions of the brain, including the likes of the hippocampus, which I assure you (because I've checked) is not a university for hippopotamus' but is the part of your noggin' that helps with mood, memory, and motivation.

As well as helping in those areas exercise helps in our abilities to distract from negative thinking and aid in social interaction. It greatly helps with our self-esteem, places barriers against our need to socially withdraw and sharpens the cognitive functions that battle against anxiety, depression, and stress.

Also, bluntly speaking, we are already aware by this point as to the side effects that come with taking antidepressants especially in terms of weight gain and the risk of obesity. Exercise is a great weapon to have in our arsenal to fight back against that.

You're not going to want to exercise at the very worst of your lowest mood and your depression is going to thrive on that.

Part of the barrier to 'getting going' is that it all feels so insurmountable and huge, and like there's no point to giving it a go because the sort of stuff you'd be able to do wouldn't make any difference anyway.

But here's the truth you may not have realised:

If you've done nothing up until this point when it comes to exercise, *anything* is going to make a difference. If exercise is something you're familiar with and was a regular part of your life in whatever capacity and you've just let it fall by the wayside because of your mental health, then this is going to be very 'crayon-thick' and 'billy basic' and I apologise. I'm shooting what follows here to the folk who've not thought of exercise as having value in the fight against their mental health issues and haven't done it before or with any sort of measured *consistency*.

This is going to be entry-level 'from nothing to something' stuff.

Like with your goal setting, like with the challenges you make against negative thinking, like with everything else we've discussed so far and will discuss hereafter, we start *small*.

We start small, we move slow, and we grow upwards.

Every PT or social media fitness influencer will try and complicate the 'pot' and that doesn't help you in trying to get this whole 'exercise' thing down into a size of consideration that feels manageable or digestible.

Let me do that for you – every exercise at its basic level can be stripped for parts and moved down to its foundational 'beginning' and ultimately when that's done it reveals for all the 'noise' it can be about just these:

1. A press-up.
2. A sit-up.
3. A squat.
4. A cardio-intensive movement.

That's it.

And the best thing of all is that if we stick with the principle of always doing more than what you did before and you've never done them before, then your starting point for the first three things is *one*.

Just one.

You read that correctly: You wake up one day and you do one press-up, one sit-up and one squat. Then tomorrow you do two of each. The next day? Three.

You see where this is going, right?

You just need to build a foundational 'base' and you can do that within a week of progressively building up each day.

Remember, we're not looking at 'the other guy' and what they're doing. Whether we're at a gym or we're in the privacy of our own home, looking at what our friends are posting online or what some celebrity is showing you they're lifting with their personal trainer. We're concentrating on just us – *our* goals and *our* fights.

I'm going to go with the possibility you know *of* these exercises only by their name and have little to nothing in terms of knowledge or experience of them.

So, humour me whilst I quickly break each of them down for you:

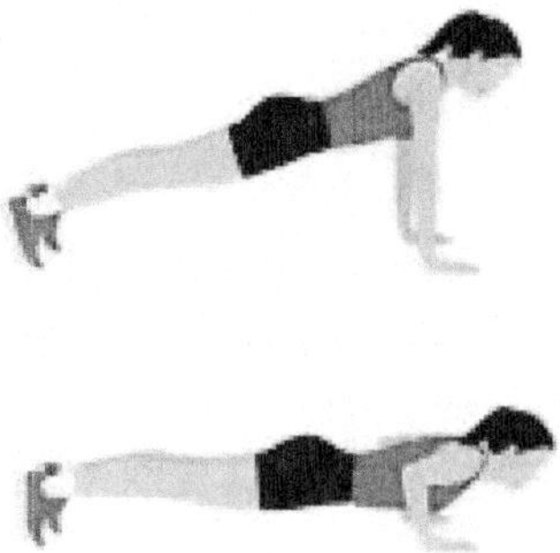

The Press-Up

The press-up remains the fundamental bodyweight exercise for working your upper-body and improving upper-body strength. It is an exercise that requires no gym equipment or gym access.

Instructions	Assistance For Starting Out
1. Lie down on the ground, get into a position where your bottom half is held up by your toes pushing into the ground and your top half is held up by your arms out straight from the ground with your hands a little wider than your shoulders. 2. Engage your body's core by holding in your stomach and lock your body into position by making sure your shoulders are pushed	To begin with you may not feel that you have the strength in your arms and across your chest to be able to affect this movement even once. Try starting out in that case by going to the stairs in your house and dropping forward onto them with your toes in position against the bottom step, get into the instructed position and push off from this angle instead. Another alternative may be to get

down away from your ears. 3. Lower your chest towards the ground with your elbows below your shoulders, creating an arrow shape with your body – the elbows representing the far corner points of the 'arrowhead'. 4. Explosively push off from the floor until you fully extend your arms. 5. Repeat this action.	into the original press-up position and then drop your knees onto the ground, so they are an additional rigid support alongside your toes. **NB:** Only use the assisted methods for the first week and then move onto unassisted each day thereafter, pushing forward daily once you have achieved your targeted goal.

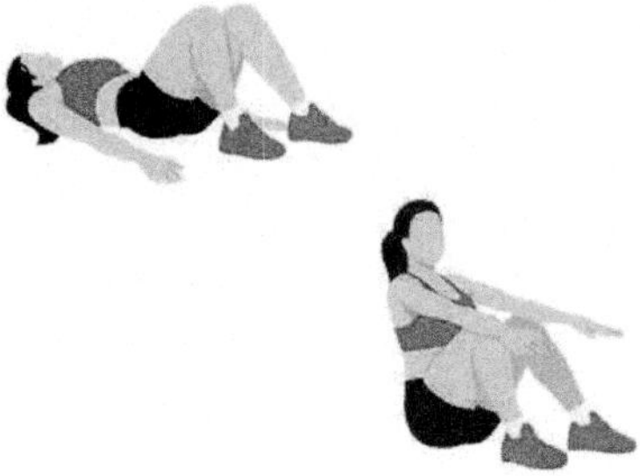

The Sit-Up

The sit-up in its most basic form is an intrinsic bodyweight exercise for working your stomach and strengthening your core. It is an exercise that requires no gym equipment or gym access.

Instructions	Assistance For Starting Out
1. Get down on the floor with your legs bent and your soles on the floor. To assist with stability throughout the exercise when starting out, feel free to tuck your feet underneath something slightly heavy (a sofa or bed) to 'pin' them. 2. Lie with your hands behind your head or straight up in front of you. Push your back into the floor and look up at the ceiling, keeping your	If a full 'extension' (i.e. from floor to the point of "crunch" where your chest meets your knees and back down again) is too much you can start by having your legs bent and in the air like an insect that has been tipped over and then simply 'crunch' your abdominals by moving the top half of your chest off the ground. Alternatively, you can do the sit-up into a 'resting stop' (i.e. let your back go flat to the ground, take a

head in a position where your chin isn't tucked into your chest, or your head isn't tilted too far back. 3. Tense your stomach and try to lift yourself all the way up so you are bringing your chest to your knees. 4. Reverse the move slowly back to the floor. Try not to go all the way down to the 'start' again. Push back to sitting up again when you feel tension in your stomach.	second to let your stomach muscles relax) and then go again. **NB:** Only use the assisted methods for the first week and then move onto unassisted each day thereafter, pushing forward daily once you have achieved your targeted goal.

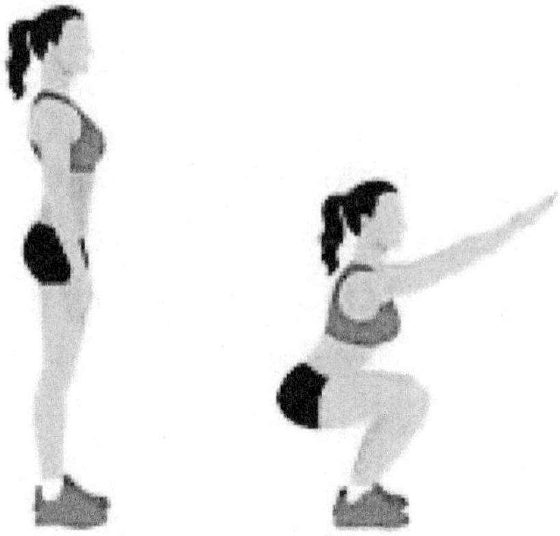

The Squat

The squat is the best of the leg exercises and helps challenge and develop improvement over other joints like the hip and the knee as well improving stability. It is an exercise that requires no gym equipment or gym access.

Instructions	Assistance For Starting Out
1. Stand with your feet a little wider than your hips. 2. Keep your chest puffed out and your stomach tight. 3. Let your hips drop back and descend whilst your knees fall in line with your toes. 4. The thighs should lower and your elbows should come in between your knees.	If you have mobility issues or are just starting out doing this exercise, concentrate on 'form' instead of 'going deep'. Drop your knees until you are at 90 degrees and have a seat behind you as a 'safety net' but only allow your bum to touch it slightly before powering back up into the starting position. **NB:** Only use the assisted methods for the first week and then move

Drive up, through the heels and tense your bum at the top as your legs straighten.	onto unassisted, pushing forward daily once you have achieved your targeted goal.

The cardio-intensive movement is very simply... *movement*! It can be whatever you feel comfortable doing, just do it for a measured amount of time that you can then build off the next day and then the next.

You can step up and down in front of the television for three to five minutes as a start. Ski slide from a side to side position whilst facing forward. Or eventually work up towards doing 'Jumping Jacks' (which are way more intense cardio-wise than you probably remember from your school days).

Remember that, medically speaking, thirty minutes of exercise of moderate intensity - brisk walking for three days a week, for example - is sufficient to be able to see the benefits of improved emotional well-being as well as the potentials for weight-loss as part of a calorie measured diet.

Best of all, the thirty minutes have been found not to need to be continuous, which means you could feasibly go for three short ten minute walks at the start, middle and end of your day and still reap the same benefits.

It's just about getting moving and then the next time moving a little bit further for a little bit longer. Sorry to drive it home again, but it is absolutely about starting small.

Keep in mind that the goal here is to work towards taking control of your mental health with exercise as one of the tools to assist – not to go out next week and take part in a 5k park run. Though that's certainly a terrific SMART goal to get working towards.

Eventually we want to get ourselves into a position where we can build what's called a 'circuit' out of these exercises and the cardio-intensive movement.

The 'circuit' is made up of 'sets' and 'reps' but that's what we work towards, yes? We start *small...*

After a week of building upwards daily we then work in our sets and reps.

A 'rep' is short for "repetition", and it is the execution of a given exercise several times over.

The 'set' is the number of times that we do that repetition to achieve our goal.

For example, if we want to achieve a goal of ten press-ups, we may do five sets of two reps broken up into a pace that is manageable to us.

It is about what you feel comfortable with, and it is important that you are always challenging and pushing yourself to work that little bit harder each time, but I advise that you only ever move on and upwards when you have successfully achieved the goal itself not because it's the next day and you're meant to.

If you're following me so far than you'll know to be trying these exercises with an increase of one each day. But if you get to Wednesday and you still can't manage three press-ups, you don't shoot for four on Thursday. You stick at achieving three and then you move on when you're ready, not because it is a specific day of the week.

A good starting point into the world of reps and sets once you've laid down your week of foundational build is to go with something that is realistic but also a challenge.

I would advocate three sets of five reps of each of the exercises with a break of sixty seconds between each set:

Exercise	Sets	Reps
Press-Ups	3	5
Sit-Ups	3	5
Squats	3	5

... You would complete five press-ups, wait sixty seconds, complete five sit-ups, wait sixty seconds, complete five squats, wait sixty seconds and then repeat all those two further times.

Then you've completed a circuit, you see?

And you've just done **fifteen** press-ups / sit-ups / squats! How cool is that?

Doing these three to five times a week will help you see the benefits mentally and emotionally. The following week, increase your reps to six. The week after that, to seven and so on.

Once you get to twelve reps, drop the reps to eight, add an additional set and go back to increasing the reps one a week:

Exercise	Sets	Reps
Press-Ups	4	8
Sit-Ups	4	8
Squats	4	8

By introducing exercise, no matter how small, into your life with consistency – measured consistency with progression as an imperative factor – you will see and feel benefits.

It kills me to have to get behind this 'rumour' regarding exercise being good for you just as much as it destroys me a little bit inside to have to acknowledge that my high school form tutor was right about how useful SMART targeting is, but it *is* true.

I still have a weird relationship with exercise in a non-competitive capacity but over the years I have found that the benefits of using it as a tool to control my mental health is almost impossible to argue against.

Exercise is a fuel that helps the 'engine' we are firing up to outrun our 'black cloud'. It tires us which improves our sleep, which in turns reduces our tiredness and increases our mental alertness and our emotional regulation...

... which helps us battle stress and feelings of anxiety. It also helps with our esteem because it helps with our weight control, which makes us feel better in ourselves and more interested in engaging socially.

"I Feel Seen" #4

THE LIFE AQUATIC WITH STEVE ZISSOU

Wes Anderson's fourth feature film remains one of his least liked, seemingly. Which is odd to me but maybe that's because it is one of my favourites of his. I take a lot of heat from people for admitting this out loud, but I prefer it to what some folk still regard to be his masterpiece, The Royal Tenenbaums. Don't get me wrong, I love The Royal Tenenbaums a lot, but it wouldn't lead the pack of my favourites of Anderson's work like this, Rushmore (another movie of Anderson's that is very nearly as autobiographical to me as Todd Solondz' Welcome To The Dollhouse), The Grand Budapest Hotel (quite possibly the man's *true* masterpiece) and Moonrise Kingdom.

I do wonder whether my love for this film is coloured by my personal attachment to it though, but more on that in a minute.

Perhaps people's difficulty to connect with this film lies with the fact Anderson's created his most unlikable of protagonists – and that's saying a lot for anyone who has seen The Royal Tenenbaums and Gene Hackman's portrayal of the lead at the centre of that film. Here Bill Murray (superbly) plays a selfish, egotistical blowhard with sociopathic tendencies and Anderson is not necessarily in a rush to redeem the character even slightly, as he did with Hackman's.

Critics were not kind at the time of The Life Aquatic With Steve Zissou's release.

The New Yorker's Anthony Lane, for example, described it as having...

"... deliberately weird set ups, which leave the viewer with the impression of having nearly drowned in some secret and melancholy game."

The film was a flop, not helped by that title admittedly. But a number of people have come round to its brilliance in the last few years, and it has been reappraised as a cult classic.

Murray plays the Steve Zissou of the film's title, a barely tolerable and eccentric oceanographer of some repute – designed in homage to the legendary French diving pioneer Jacques Cousteau (to which Anderson dedicates this film) – who has devoted his next expedition, what little finances he has left and the safety of his crew to tracking down and killing a 'jaguar shark' that ate his diving / business partner, Esteban. All whilst trying to deal with the arrival of a journalist (Cate Blanchett) out to cover his trail of vengeance, the son he didn't know he had (Owen Wilson), business rivals (Jeff Goldblum) and an assortment of issues with his crew (most memorably represented by an overly sensitive member of staff brilliantly portrayed by a very funny Willem Dafoe).

Anderson has made a beautiful-looking film, and he doesn't get enough credit for that, if nothing else. It also contains one of the best performances Bill Murray has ever given us; it's very funny in an acerbically dry way and he makes us want to spend time within this film's narrative with a character that we would otherwise find far too abrasive to pass five minutes in the company of in real life.

Steve Zissou:

"Now if you'll excuse me, I'm going to go on an overnight drunk, and in 10 days I'm going to set out to find the shark that ate my friend and destroy it. Anyone who wants to tag along is more than welcome."

It’s eminently quotable (“That's an endangered species at most. What would be the scientific purpose of killing it?” “Revenge.”) and what's more, tucked away inside of it is a sequence involving the assault on the pirates' hide-out that answers the question as to what a "*Wes Anderson Action Movie*" would look like - and it would look extremely good indeed!

If you've never experienced this, you owe it to yourself to. It's most certainly not broad comedy but it proves to hit the comedic marks it wants to - and it's surprisingly and profoundly *moving* too!

How moving?

Well, let’s deal in **spoilers** for a twenty-ish year old movie here:

In the finale Anderson and Murray deliver a moment / denouement that didn’t land with me on first viewing but then suddenly hit me like a wrecking ball a couple of years later and helped change my life.

At the film’s end, Zissou finally tracks down this almost mythical ‘jaguar shark’ in his submersible surrounded by his key crew and what could at best be considered his family (an ex-wife played by Anjelica Huston) but can’t bring himself to kill it even though doing so is all that has driven him in the time we’ve spent with the character.

He is overcome by its visual beauty (and the fact he is out of dynamite!) and suddenly breaks down with emotion, simply stating "I wonder if it remembers me?" as those around him gently put their hand on him to provide comfort.

Once consumed by a vengeful anger (and the egotism of believing that a recording of his pursuit would be a boon for his waning career), Zissou simply lets the creature go and, in the process, let’s go of the thirst for retribution that was driving him.

By the time I hit my mid-thirties and I’d go so far as to say even at the point I was exiting out of them and going into my forties, I was entrenched with anger myself.

I’d let go of *nothing* except the trauma of my military days that had eventually drove me to be diagnosed with PTSD and receive treatment.

Now, if you measured me up against my ability to move on from what I experienced there, how I ruminated about it, the guilt I felt and so forth than I would present as a picture of strong mental health and a poster child for robust coping mechanisms in this regard...

... but the *reality* outside of this was decidedly different; I was beaten down by the repeated failure to 'beat' my depression once and for all even after this successful PTSD treatment, I could not understand why my relationships with those around me were so routinely awkward and upsetting and I felt there had to be something wrong with me if no one including my own family liked me.

I started to carry an extreme grudge about how every attempt I made to move forward was met with a knock-back whilst those around me cheated, lied, back-stabbed and moved forward in my place without any negative recourse upon them.

I hated myself. I hated my life. I was newly married and starting a family and every day I would start each day wondering if today was the day my wife was going to 'see sense' and leave me or I was going to fuck something up that harmed my newborn child like I messed everything else up.

I could not get my head around why anyone would want to be with someone like me. You know that whole 'You have to love yourself before anyone can love you' nonsense?

Well, I abjectly *hated* myself and my life and I started to think less of those around me for seeing good in me. Woody Allen did this great gag ("I'd never join a club that would allow a person like me to become a member.") and I used to look at what friends I had, my wife, etc and I used to push myself to think "I don't think I want to associate with the sort of people that think highly or like me because I am bloody awful."

I was desperate to be liked and to be accepted as part of some sort of personal validation and yet I was driving away anyone who liked or accepted me for me because I thought there must be something wrong with them for doing so.

That's something that Carl Jung would have had a field day with, huh? My baseline foundation lay with me telling myself that if my own family didn't even like me why would / should anyone else?

It was very easy to build a whole skyscraper of negativity off the back of that and I did too. And then I piled the injustices I experienced on top of that as well, and my inability to process them and let go of them deeply affected me.

I came to work in a role within 'uniformed services' in my later life through the ego-boost of them coming to me and headhunting me to apply.

They'd seen work I had done elsewhere in my particular field (some that had reflected poorly on them by the time matters had gone before the courts) and it seemed a bit like 'better the devil you know' in them bringing me in to do what I was doing anyway but *for* them.

It proved to be a terrible mistake on my part.

Once in the job I realised I was surrounded by colleagues that put me in an ethical minefield – this was a public body wholly built upon honesty, integrity, lawfulness and civic trust.

Yet a large volume of people I worked with on a day-to-day basis were inherently dishonest, prejudiced and sometimes downright criminal and hateful in their conduct towards the public they served.

The staff who weren't were routinely fighting an uphill battle to stay sane or, at minimum, professionally progress. I became one of them.

I saw all the posters in the staff changing room and around the corridors about speaking out and challenging unprofessional conduct and inappropriateness, especially at a time when the public's confidence (rightly) was at an all-time low for this particular uniformed service.

When I saw one of my younger female colleagues carry out a sex act on another member of staff on the organisation's premises then later brag about that person helping her cheat on a formal exam, I reported it.

I didn't report it for the purposes of trying to hobble her or get her in trouble as a matter of priority.

I reported it because she openly bragged about it in an office with me present and I was genuinely worried that if it was investigated and I was found to have witnessed it and not reported it I could be in just as much trouble... that's what all the posters around the station were warning anyway.

Doing so brought me to a place of professional detriment. I'll not relitigate it from my earlier recounting of it.

But what was worse for me was finding out that whilst I was 'frozen' from professional development and advancement going forward (often with superiors purposefully and maliciously altering achievement possibilities for me just as I was reaching them, all to prevent me from 'getting there'), they handed everything on a platter to the younger female colleague despite her reputation for, quote unquote, "the worst ineptitude this job has ever seen" according to one boss. I challenged the fairness in what was occurring to me and was told by one senior manager "She fucks people who can benefit her. Are you going to start fucking people? Because you're a bit too old, out of shape and you've left it too late to even think about it, if you ask me!"

The blatant corruption and injustice hit me, and it completely took over me. I could not believe it was happening and being allowed to happen.

What's more, honest and hardworking colleagues of mine started leaking information about what was going on inside the organisation to the press and they were met with the same response again and again:

'Oh, that's typical of [Named Public Body]. They've had a problem with the toxic culture in there forever. That's never going to change, everyone knows that. That's why it's not newsworthy.'

My colleagues couldn't believe it. I couldn't either. But they could shrug it off and move on.

I couldn't.

I took it and I ate it up and mentally drowned myself in the unfairness, the dishonesty, and the immorality of what was meant to be a trusted public body.

I would sit up all night thinking and overthinking. I would drink heavily. I would write huge long emails full of evidence as to the illegality or the discrimination I was facing.

I would even have managers try and pull me back from the brink by meeting me for coffee informally outside of work and advising me to 'leave it alone' because the colleague in question had an affair with an influential superintendent and "there's connections at play there now you don't want to mess with", apparently.

My anger didn't abate. The injustice didn't go away.

Colleagues would try and diminish what was going on by simply saying "This shit is the way it's always been around here. Only the people change."

It didn't make a difference. I don't know why I ever expected a different outcome – that hard work would be rewarded accordingly, that honesty and integrity would be valued in an organisation where those characteristics are imperative – when it had not been my experience up to that point. This one thing was the 'straw' and I was the 'camel's back'.

I should have been able to let it go.

I wanted to be able to let it go. I couldn't.

I simply drove everyone around me crazy, relitigating the unfairness and telling all and sundry about the mounds of corruption and dishonesty I was a witness to inside of an organisation they stupidly hold too much trust in.

I'd tell the 'Gorillas in a Cage' fable again and again to whoever I was speaking to and then one day I caught sight of my reflection in a mirror across from my table in a pub and quietly thought to myself "You look fucking insane, pal!"

You're familiar with the 'Gorillas in a Cage' fable, no?

A zoological experiment is conducted by placing five gorillas in a cage and at the centre is a banana hanging from the roof with a ladder directly beneath it.

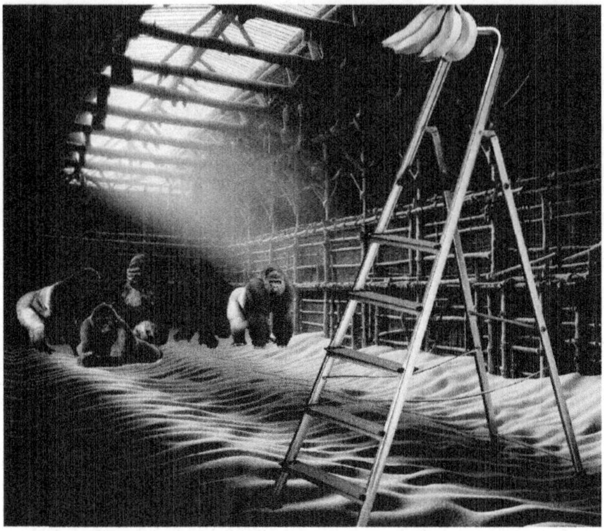

As one of the gorillas begins to climb the ladder toward the banana, a zookeeper sprays all five gorillas with a fire hose full of cold water. The gorillas scatter. A few hours pass and one of the gorillas goes to approach the ladder again, the hose comes on and they all get sprayed again.

The next day one of the gorillas tentatively tiptoes towards the ladder but is stopped by the other four who do not want to be hit with the water. One of the gorillas is removed from the cage that day and replaced with a new one. The new gorilla obviously goes for the banana but is instantly attacked by the others.

Soon a second is removed and replaced with a new one. Same thing happens – banana / ladder is approached, an attack occurs. No explanation is provided as to why.

A third gorilla is replaced, and the same events occur.

Eventually, the last two original gorillas cowering in the corner are swapped and now the cage is filled with five gorillas with no knowledge of why they should not approach the ladder, will never touch the ladder, or ever get their hands on that delicious looking banana.

One day one of the gorillas turns to the others and says “Hey, I’ve been thinking – why don’t I go get that banana and we’ll all share it.” The others all reply “No! No!” and “Don’t touch the banana!” He asks why and the reply is “Because that’s the way it’s always been around here.”

For me, it is the greatest allegory to explain how corruption builds without ever getting dented or put a stop to and how dishonest and undeserved people prosper in those sorts of environments.

Go along with the status quo, no matter how fucked it is.

Stick with the group and don’t express any individual thought. Turn a blind eye... and you’ll be alright!

To put it plainly, I broke myself.

I allowed myself to lose control of some of the more burgeoning tactics I had started to formulate around control over my mental health, especially when it had come to processing childhood abuse and self-esteem.

I simply crumbled under the heavy weight of the injustice and the helpless feeling of being victim to such corrupt conduct by figures meant to be acting with the utmost integrity.

There’s a whole other discussion to come later regarding my eventual mental collapse and the road that formed out of it to lead towards writing this book.

But one move in the right direction towards a healthier outlook with me at the helm of my own emotional wellbeing was a drunken, late night viewing of The Life Aquatic With Steve Zissou and upon hearing that "I wonder if it remembers me?" something in me *released...*

Not one single instigator of my happiest feelings was in any way attached to that job within that organisation.

Not one person who I valued or considered a friend from my experience working there felt any differently than what I did about the circumstances surrounding that colleague, their conduct, or the toxic work environment they thrived in.

I drew no value from doing the job and progression within it was something that I looked at as a means of escape not as something I necessarily wanted to do.

I had received professional commendations and achievements within my field on an international level, but they were all from my time *prior* to joining this organisation.

So, why in that case was I allowing this job with this uniformed service to have such a hold on me?

You know that friend I mentioned earlier in 'The Cost of a Text'? Well, very early on within my mental anguish over this whole saga, he asked me "If they made you redundant tomorrow, outside of the hassle that comes with having to find another job, would you actually care?" and I realised that I didn't.

I didn't respect that organisation and the dishonest way they held power over the community they were meant to serve any more than I respected my parents for the way they had raised me as if I was a 'lesser' person of value because of my interests, hobbies, or outlook.

I had been able to reach a point of healthily cutting my parents from my life for the good of my mental health and the wellbeing of my family going forward. Why couldn't I simply do that with my involvement with this job I was employed in?

Why was I *allowing* them to have power over me like this?

They were undeserved of it.

And right there, in that moment watching the conclusion of The Life Aquatic With Steve Zissou as he premieres his finished documentary and receives a standing ovation, I realised that this job was completely *undeserving* of me. I had value and I had dignity, neither of which I wanted to allow them to have another chance to abuse or take advantage of.

I breathed out at the realisation that I was in control, not them.

As a result, I let go of the anger that was derailing my ability to move forward.

Removing The Tumour:

Self-Surgery / Proactive Problem Solving

Strap yourselves in, folks. We're going to go *deep*.

The simple truth is that to best outpace our mental health issues or to succeed in our goals it is an impossibility to do so without looking inwards at yourself and getting reflective.

And there's a very strong chance when you do that some of your negative thought will carry actual weight because there's evidence / facts there to support it or there's elements of your life now jumping out at you as being a harmful or adverse impactor that you know has got to change for you to be able to progress and develop.

You could be experiencing low mood because of the loss of a dear friendship, which hypothetically has ended due to your friend deeming you to be selfish.

Such an accusation hurts and offends, obviously. Especially because of the impact it has had on the friendship.

But what if you were to take a second and put that under the spotlight like we discussed earlier around catastrophic thinking – do you put your own needs first a lot of the time, are you only getting in touch or being proactive with your contact when *you* have an issue...

If you start to realise that there's been incidents of such behaviour it is important to maintain the perspective that you've behaved in such a way but that doesn't mean that's *who you are* as a person overall. You can then take ownership of it and address it.

It is unhelpful for you, your mental health, and your future personal development if you reflect, see the evidence, not like it, and try and deflect with a whole heap of "Yeah but..."

It's even worse if you take hold of the thought and allow it to overcome you, define you and take control of you emotionally. More on that in a minute though.

If you were to draw up a table right now with four columns on it, covering life, love, work and finances and you had to assess your state of happiness with regards to each would they sit blank because you're happy with where you are at in each of them or would you have to bullet-point *some* things for each? What would they be?

Have you ever asked yourself that directly or have you been anxious around what you might unpick from doing it, so you've just buried it all instead?

When it comes to our love lives, this is apparently incredibly common. We aren't happy and we're not fulfilled within the relationship, but we sigh, and we think about the shared rent / mortgage, the children, or the dog and how awkward it will be to split all that. We think about shitty companionship being better than no company at all because our self-worth is that low. And we simply accept our lot in this element of our life as being all we're deserved of, instead of looking inwards at what's not working and getting reflective as to why.

Be bold. Be brave. Try it:

Life	Love	Career	Financial

We spend too much time thinking that things have got to change without ever proactively engaging in anything to *affect* change.

We want more money for example, but we don't chase the jobs in our field of expertise that offer it elsewhere from our current employer. Predominantly we wait where we are and hope for promotions or natural wage increases instead.

In my late twenties I looked inwards for the first time at who I was to try and figure out why I was experiencing the things in life I was and why my interactions with other people were often so fruitless in terms of value.

My problem was I didn't have the mental or emotional maturity and experience at that point in my life to process what I felt I discovered in a healthy way. Instead, I just let it consume me and take over my life and it came to affect my mental health in an even more corrosive way.

What I did realise then was something I couldn't recognise the magnitude of until much later in my life – that I was allowing too much of my life and my personality to be defined or controlled by other people or my need to have their approval, which is dangerous in many ways but all the more so if the people in question are not deserved of it or have toxic traits / outlooks that are pushed or projected upon you. Nowadays I use the 'Tigger' analogy:

When I was a small child one of my teachers gave me the nickname of 'Tigger'. As she described it, I was continually enthusiastic and always looking for the bright side of a given situation whilst trying to cheer up anyone who was feeling down.

A great personality to have as a kid, right?

God, *yeah*!

I'm very pleased to say that both of my children are 'Tigger' kids and I fully and actively endorse it.

But with me, in time, other kids polluted the nickname, and it was no longer attributed to me in a positive way.

I was joked about as someone who "never shut up" and was "always bouncing around, annoying everyone". Before I'd even hit ten years of age this nickname that once made me glow and smile when the teacher called me it turned into a 'label' I would react angrily to if it was used.

I'd allowed other people to take control of something I enjoyed and something that made me feel positive, and I'd let them twist it into something else so they could use it to hurt me or feel bad.

It was something that would course through the rest of my life for quite some time thereafter in different permutations.

I'd went from seeing myself as someone who was 'enthusiastic' about being in your company to, at far too young an age, seeing myself as the 'irritant' around you.

And I owned that when I shouldn't have, I think.

I spent so long failing to recognise that I was not purposefully an annoyance, but a child raised without worth who was just desperate to be your friend, eager to be accepted or loved. Or desirous to feel that I had *value*.

I once read that the best thing you can do if you're about to be attacked by a wolf is to piss your pants because allegedly the stench of urine is so repulsive to them that they will run from it.

There's a lot of bullshit out there on the internet.

This is *likely* to be some of it. I don't know.

(I remember once reading about a guy who said if a pitbull locked its jaws on you then you should insert a finger into its anus as the pressure on its gland will cause the jaw to relax. I totally bought that without question first and queried what the hell he was doing at the time to discover *that* unfortunately second!)

I *do* think there's something to this in humans when it comes to the smell of *desperation* though. People smelt how desperate I was to be loved and accepted and they fled from it or exploited it in horrible and cruel ways.

I remember one time – the end of June 1993, to be exact because no amount of counselling has helped in forgetting it – at the height of the worst period of being bullied at school, two of the more popular kids came over and asked if I wanted to go and see Cliffhanger with them that weekend.

I was guarded and suspicious at first because why would these kids be interested in hanging out with me – especially outside of school seeing as they didn't give me the time of day *in* school. They assured me they wanted to 'start' being my friend, they felt sorry for me apparently and I bought it.

I was *that* desperate to be liked and valued I believed them.

I was so excited for Saturday afternoon, more so because I was so hungry to see Cliffhanger (people forget these days but the marketing and promotion for that film was nothing short of exquisite back then!) equal to finally being 'accepted'.

I spent the rest of the week talking to my grandma about the upcoming cinema trip and how "cool" these other kids were, and I showed up outside the old Odeon twenty minutes early just to be sure.

They were late… then they were late enough that, okay we were going to miss the adverts but hopefully not the trailers… then they were so late that they were cutting it fine for the start of the film and…

… then I saw across on the other side of the busy road they were stood laughing uproariously with my bullies, whilst pointing at me.

Out of nowhere a lad from school stepped from behind me and smashed an egg into my face then ran off to join the group. They all then jumped around laughing before disappearing off round the corner.

A lady at the bus-stop nearby came over with a handkerchief and helped me get the thick of the egg off.

I was so embarrassed.

And hurt.

I could feel the tears welling up inside.

I thanked her and went inside the Odeon to use the toilets to clean myself up properly and once I was done, I realised I was too embarrassed to go home so soon and too scared to wander around the city centre on my own in case I bumped into the kids from school.

So, I bought my ticket for Cliffhanger and my popcorn, and I went and watched the film alone. I wiped away my tears through the last couple of trailers I was able to catch and by the time that [still unbelievable] aerial stunt between the two planes was playing out on screen I wasn't thinking about what had happened to me... or the missed bit of yolk hardening in the side of my hair. Films, man. They're *powerful*, I keep telling you.

The day that I started to look back over my life and my feelings (and not just instantly take ownership for them like I was some sort of bad person or failure, but to hold them to account and fact-check or stress test them) was the day I went from being the guy who saw enough of himself in the protagonist of Midnight Run to feel inspired to change but not know how, to being the man who got far enough along to be able to recognise mental health issues are simply *in* us; foibles in our personality make us who we are and our mental health is the same. And if we can control our lesser qualities – greed, selfishness, rudeness, etc – then we can control that too.

It's all about *how*.

Even John McClane in Die Hard took a moment to get self-introspective about himself and the impact his behaviour was having on his marriage – and *he* was in the middle of getting shot at by multiple people, jumping off the top of buildings whilst tied to a fire hose and running over broken glass with no shoes on.

Yet, if you'll recall, he was still able to do a little bit of self-surgery and recognise that he'd been "a jerk" and that he'd not been as supportive to his wife when her career started to develop as he could have been.

His self-reflection led him to realise that she was the best thing that ever happened to a bum like [him] and that he needed to apologise to her.

If he can do a mental health 'MOT' like that on himself whilst fighting off robbers who are pretending to be terrorists, I think you can give it a go too, no?

One of the keyways as to how is to look at the impactors on our mental health and our relationship to as well as our control over them. The biggest statistically speaking is work and our position in the world of employment.

In getting to the position I am in now with regards to the control I feel I have over my mental health I looked back over my own career and I also spoke with friends who are struggling with stress and anxiety at work or are suffering from depression because of work related matters.

Do you know what one of the things was that became screamingly apparent as a throughline amongst all of our respective experiences and emotional detriments accrued from work?

The fact that we lost sight of our ability or our right to say, "*I'm doing the best I can!*" so long ago or so far back down the line that it's starting to seem possible we may never have had ownership of it all. How insane is that?

This applies both to our working lives and our personal lives – this feeling we imbue ourselves with that it is wrong or weak of us just to tell our partner, our family, our colleagues or our friends that we're working at full capacity and we're doing the best that we are capable of but that the problem, the situation or the feeling may actually be *more* than you and you alone are capable of dealing with.

Saying something as truly simple as "I'm doing the best I can!" to an employer who is being *unknowingly* unreasonable in their expectations of your output, work-rate, etc given the hours in the day could well yield a positive outcome for you.

But it seems we have this intrinsic fear of saying this out loud especially at work because we worry our best may be perceived as not good enough and then we're drawing attention to a professional failing.

Yet is it good enough within the actual healthy parameters of the job you're employed to do, not the job that's come to be expected of you by the people in managerial roles above you.

You see, when we get self-introspective, and we look inwards (specifically around the impactors affecting us at work) we can often see that we are doing everything required of our role but it's the factors being applied *additional* to it that we didn't ask for or shouldn't be taking on where the wheels start to come off.

Nine times out of ten this is due to someone above you removing a worry of theirs and putting it on to you because their authority allows them to.

How many times have you heard the expression 'Shit rolls downhill'? There's staff sickness in the department and the person off sick has left tasks incomplete ahead of an important deadline. The manager is very unlikely to take that work across the finish line themselves. They'll delegate it to you to fit in with the work you're trying to get done to your own deadline. Now you have twice the amount of work in the same amount of time and the manager's stress is owned by you. If / when you fail, the 'buck' stops with you as the cause of the failure because you didn't get done what needed done.

Repeatedly we apologise or we try and negotiate for more time if we're brave enough. What we never seem to do is take the expression 'Shit rolls downhill' and challenge it like it is a catastrophic thought or a feeling needing fact-checked by questioning "Why do I need to wait at the bottom of the hill though?"

When we start asking that question within the workplace we begin to possibly reflect on our situation and see that we are not being appreciated or respected. We're being seen as 'fodder' and no matter the job, we deserve better than that. We deserve to be valued and we're entitled to draw value from our day's work.

The quickest and easiest way to begin an accurate assessment regarding work and the impact it is having on you is to firstly list what worth other than financial you wish to draw from the job and then alongside it note whether you're getting it. If not, why not? It's very likely indeed that the notes you make here are going to speedily identify the stress / depression impactors work is having on your mental health.

Once you've done this, schedule a meeting with your manager(s) and raise these as welfare issues specific to how the work concerns are affecting you emotionally and mentally.

It could be that you are carrying too many people's workloads, a change in working practise has left you impacted in some way, you're not getting enough time to complete work or receive feedback on the work you're doing, or that you're being bullied or victimised in some way by colleagues.

It's important that you raise the issue because it's not so much about getting the matter on record as it is about getting a measure or feeling as to how they ***react*** to what you say.

A negative reaction, a response of indifference or punitive measures implemented is the fastest route to knowing what your value is within the organisation – and that it *isn't* good. Getting out of there to a place of respect and appreciation then becomes an immediate SMART goal for yourself, doesn't it?

One of the best pieces of advice I ever received when it comes to toxic workplaces and matters around work-related stress is this:

Let the good staff be your guiding light to the exit.

What that means is that if a work environment is unprofessional, unhealthy, and poisonous to your mental well-being you can normally tell because the good employees leave.

They know that they're too good to have to put up with this.

The people that usually follow them out the door are the employees who thought they could change things for the better but got burdened down with the stress.

Usually the stress of trying to complete their own workload plus carrying the work of all those good people that have left.

What is now left are the people that are causing the problems in the first place alongside the people that feel they are 'tied' there because of their age, circumstances or because they've been dumped in this department due to behavioural concerns (the department in the uniformed service I worked in was absolutely *rife* with staff members who hadn't hit the threshold of being sackable but needed to be 'contained' all the same).

What I have come to realise the older I have got and the more I have prioritised my mental health is that there is greater personal value in spotting the unprofessional, unhealthy, and poisonous environment and *getting out of there* than there is in suffering personal detriment trying to change something you cannot.

Challenging or shutting down the stress at work can often turn out to be a very positive impacting thing. If your approach to doing so is respectful and professional. The moment I decided I was going to bring the "I'm doing the best I can!" mantra into my working life, the changes were seismic. It helped put barriers up against stresses, it spotlighted where my value was within the organisation and who with. It really made me see clearly that my role was to carry additional responsibilities of middle-managers who didn't want the work themselves and that the welfare impact on me was utterly immaterial to them.

This last point is *imperative* in making you establish your worth and separate yourself from a job that is making you ill.

How often have we heard the term 'burn out' used in the workplace?

The jobs that see 'burn out' in staff emerging off in the distance and don't do anything to stop it before it grows or lands?

The job that sees employees as to be worked to 'burn out' and then replaced with 'fresh' staff?

Those are the jobs you *don't* want.

Why is your current organisations' profit margins or positive workflow statistics more important than your emotional wellbeing?

These sort of jobs - if you want to hold control of your mental health and stay ahead of your 'black cloud' - <u>must</u> get replaced as a matter of urgency.

We should all take time to look inwards at ourselves and do what I call a little bit of a 'Mental MOT' for the good of our emotional health and it's important that we are robust but fair with ourselves. We should be direct and honest about our feelings and where they're coming from, but we should also be tender and forgiving too.

We must be cautious not to look for scapegoats though. In looking inwards at myself and really trying to get to a place of understanding, if not acceptance, about why I appeared to always be an easy target for bullying or exploitation from people and why I seemed to be found to be so irritating and / or disagreeable in the eyes of people within a quick amount of time it was all too easy for me to hide behind the same thought again and again:

"I'm too eager to be accepted and this comes from a lack of self-worth, which is because of my abusive upbringing and the lack of strong emotional foundations I was raised with – so it's my parents fault and I will never forgive them for this because now I'm damaged goods!"

The reality is that at the point of getting to an interesting and sincere point of reflection about myself, I put the blame at someone else's door and locked it off as a stringent 'fact' that defines who I am and did nothing worthwhile with it. It negated the reason and the value in doing a bit of 'self-surgery' on myself in the first place.

Rather than leave it on the proverbial 'doorstep' of my parents, I challenged the catastrophic thinking elements of the drawn thought and held it up to an evidential spotlight:

I *was* damaged by the absence of worth and respect I was raised with but who is to say that this damage is permanent? If it's not permanent than it can be changed or improved upon, but how?

Well, we challenge ourselves a little further to get more detailed answers in this case.

Now, in my case I looked at where I was drawing my feelings of self-confidence and personal value from, and I asked myself why I'm putting something as important and powerful as this in the hands of *other people*.

As an adult now with all the responsibilities, tribulations, benefits, and handicaps that come with that, why was I refusing to chase dreams or ambitions because they're not the dreams or ambitions my parents told me I should have? Why was I pushing to be accepted by colleagues whose integrity and professionalism was below the level of what I feel is important or proper, simply because I wanted to be included in the 'small talk' that they indulged in throughout the day or the afterwork drinks that they covertly arranged when they thought I wasn't listening?

One day, whilst carrying out this 'self-surgery' thing I got to thinking about why I was chasing the veneration of colleagues that I wouldn't associate with or consider as friends outside of work.

"You're chasing an invite to a gathering you wouldn't go to even if you got it," I said to myself. It was a small enough mental confrontation for me to push forward as to why I was chasing the respect of people *I* didn't respect... which was a huge boon on staring down the issues I had with my family:

Why does the thoughts and opinions of people I don't like nor think a lot of hold weight with me? Why should it? It shouldn't. So, what am I going to do about that?

That line of self-reflection for me and the line of thought I drew from it (to get to a place where I realised that my desperation to please and be liked was all from basing my personal value on what other people thought of me) was a complete game-changer in my life and in my ability to get down the right path towards taking control of my mental health.

Going back to the work / welfare situation, I took this new line of thought about my own value into my place of employment within the uniformed services.

I realised that every time extra duty, complicated jobs and thankless tasks were needing done I was stepping up instantly as standard to take them on because I thought it would ingratiate me with my team-mates and make them like me more.

It didn't.

I ended up in no greater a position of esteem with them but simply with a far greater amount of work and stress, as well as a developed reputation and expectation that I was the 'soft touch' who would do this all the time, so they didn't have to.

Then one day with my new line of thought about self-respect I simply asked myself "What if I didn't? What if my hand didn't go up first? I'm at no risk of a loss of their respect and affection towards me because I don't have it anyway..."

And that day I didn't step up first and foremost for 'the shit task'.

The request hung in the air.

My colleagues looked at me.

I looked round at each of them.

My manager eyeballed me, waiting for me to speak.

I didn't.

They picked another begrudging member of staff instead and the machinations of the day moved forward once more regardless, only this time with me a little bit less stressed out than I otherwise would have been.

It doesn't need to be complicated. There need be no overt confrontation of any aggressive nature, with yourself or anyone else.

You merely look at yourself. You register what it is you don't like, or you think could be contributing negatively. You ask yourself how you could change that. You make a proactive move towards changing it.

That's it. That's all it is. Lay it out in writing for yourself. I think you'll be surprised in yourself by what you read back:

What is a situation in your life that is making you think or feel negatively about yourself?	
What is the negative feeling you are experiencing and why do you think you are feeling this way?	
How could you change this feeling in yourself or what do you think would have to change?	
What one small SMART goal could you set yourself that would proactively effect a change in this feeling you have	

or the situation you're experiencing?	

Researchers from the University of California Berkeley published a study in the April 2024 edition of Behaviour Research and Therapy regarding how positive affirmations boosted mental health, and mental wellbeing in turn improved considerably the more often such affirmations were carried out.

They claim speaking kindly to yourself for even less than a minute a day could benefit your emotional and mental state.

They tested 100 people to assess whether 'self-compassionate touch' (steady now, perverts!), which involves placing your hands on your chest and repeating statements like 'How can I be a friend to myself at this moment' could improve mental health.

Participants were asked to practice the exercises for at least 20 seconds every day for one month. The results indicated that those who carried out these exercises reduced their stress levels, improved their emotional well-being, and gained greater self-compassion.

Now, I vowed at the start of this book we weren't going to do the inspirational quotes thing and I'll be damned if we're going to start now.

Nor am I suggesting that you need to start doing 'self-affirmations' in the mirror each morning. I am *so* not that guy, and I am not advocating you become that type of person either regardless of the results from the above study.

Unless that sort of thing 'floats your boat', in which case fill your boots. Remember, this is about what works for you and what you're comfortable with.

What I can tell you is that a lot of good comes from getting to the core of your negative feeling, writing a challenge against it to yourself on a post-it note and putting that note next to you bed... on top of your phone or whatever your morning alarm is.

Reading that first thing agendas it into your conscious. And it feels a little less 'hippy dippy' than standing looking at yourself in the mirror and growling or something.

My suggestion sounds trippy and silly, I know but it *works*.

Especially with simple, straight directives to yourself. They don't need to be overly emotive 'affirmations' or something that make you feel self-conscious or silly. They can just be a question that sets your mind up for the day ahead.

Routinely mine would be things like "What's one thing you would feel good about achieving today?" or "Will you be kinder to yourself today than yesterday?"

Sometimes I would write a little note to myself on the subject line of my phone's alarm setting so when the alarm went off in the morning, I would see ~~affirmations~~ statements like "Embrace the good. Challenge the bad."

They don't work as immediate laser blasts of emotional course-correction. But they *do* plant the seed you need planted within a couple of seconds of waking up to lean more positively into the day from the get-go.

Wearing Your Wounds

One of the words I kept hearing time and again by friends and therapists to describe me was resilient. I used to brace against it. "Oh, you've been through so much. I don't know how you're still standing. You're so resilient." For the longest time I just used to feel that it was a word they fell back on to use because they didn't know what to say to all the abuse I've described or bullying I've endured, or opportunities I've blown by displaying an objectionable personality and desperately trying too hard. I felt like they awkwardly tried to commend me rather than judge or counsel me and the best that they could come up with was 'resilient'.

The greater an understanding I gained over my own mental health (and with it a sense of *control* – that term again!) and the older I got the more I started to see value in being described as 'resilient'. Suddenly the word didn't feel like a 'buffer' description but a one that captured my ability to stay ahead of my ol' black cloud, to have the fortitude to recognise it gaining in speed on some days and to still be able to outpace it - I've been abused, I've been bullied, I've been professionally hobbled for not 'playing the game', I've had monumental personal and work-related set-backs at times (sometimes when I've been my own worst enemy), I've had breakdowns, breakthroughs and suicide attempts... and I've endured and came out the other side *a little less* bitter than I once was but with a strong desire to help others through to the lighter side too.

I'm the hare.

The hare was resilient.

I'm *okay* with resilient now.

The shift came first with that 'self-surgery' we looked at a couple of chapters back. The more I scrutinised myself the more I started to realise that there was a hole in me that I wouldn't allow to be filled. It could have been filled easily. But I objected to what it was filled with. This is not the time for innuendo. There was an emptiness inside of me. I kept seeking this validation, this feeling of being exceptional at... *something*! And it had existed inside of me for so long that it had taken over my personality. I didn't put it there. My parents did at the youngest possible age, and it grew out of control – this notion that I *must* be exceptional, or I *must* achieve 'A' and earn 'B' or do 'C' or I would not be deserved of love and respect.

Taking that and dropping it / exorcising it, which wasn't easy and took time and ultimately cutting my parents from my life once and for all, caused an altering of perspective that helped with the second shift; accepting that as we age, physically and mentally, our perceptions and intentions shift in many ways especially emotionally. We see things differently and we *should* see them differently too but also, we want different things. Sometimes all too often we lie to ourselves about this or deny ourselves access to them out of a worry what others may think or what impact chasing then acquiring them will have on our life as it is right at that moment.

In my opinion we spend our childhood and our teenage years looking around us at what other kids our age are into and it's all too common that we align ourselves with what the majority think is "cool" because we want to fit in.

By the time we hit our twenties we are facing down this sudden wall of expectation from all and sundry about what we are going to do with our lives now we're "grown up" when all the while we're secretly thinking "I'm only just figuring out what it is *I* actually like because I spent the last five to ten years liking some shit my friends told me was great or doing something everyone else was doing..."

We arrive in our thirties feeling like we tripped and fell into them, the job we got whilst we were trying to 'figure out' what we wanted to do is now our career and we're acting as connective tissue between our childhood friends, the 'friends' we now have because we spend eight to ten hours a day and five days a week with them and the friends that are emerging through us embracing the things we truly enjoy.

Then you age into the over forties demographic and suddenly you start to understand yourself more than you ever have and become comfortable in just liking what you like, and valuing what you utilise your time on.

I look back now and realise that people's perception of the life I have lived was a valuable indicator in marking the shift as I aged. By the end of my twenties people used to act so awed as I talked about my life over the last decade – the varied jobs I've done, the countries I've lived in, the crazy anecdotes and injuries I'd amassed. By the end of my thirties there was no awe, more a lot of questions about what it was I was seemingly running from and what toll such injuries and antics had taken on me. A person's perspective can evolve of you over time. It's only logical that your own perspective of yourself can do the same thing.

There's a great moment in that Billy Crystal comedy City Slickers. His character, Mitch Robbins, attends his young son's career day to give a talk to the class but his emotional crisis gets the better of him and he ends up doing this extended comedic monologue about valuing life because it goes by so quickly. Check the film out anyway, it's a classic. But that scene alone is a real *beaut'* for what we're talking about in this chapter.

The more in control of your mental health you become, especially in terms of coming to understand what triggers severe or profound negative emotional feeling, the more you come to value and appreciate what you like and what you are comfortable with because of the benefits they offer. And with that, letting go of the things that you don't like or only ever felt pressure to take part in.

Imperatively, it is important to embrace the things you like because you like them and that's *enough.* That moment when you move away from the period in your teenage years when you pretended your favourite author was Bret Easton Ellis (or Jonathan Safran Foer in your late twenties to make yourself appear more sensitive than you were), to simply saying "I like Dennis LeHane, Elmore Leonard and Judy Blume, Goddamnit. And I've *always* liked them and *just* them!" is a seismic moment. It represents more than you realise.

Let me put it into one of those movie analogies you'll have come to expect of me by now – Have you heard of that movie, Bird on a Wire? The 1990 John Badham action comedy with Mel Gibson and Goldie Hawn about a guy in the Witness Protection programme who must go on the run across America with this ex-lover when the villains from his past track him down? Well, I like that movie a lot.

If you go off critical consensus from around its release and the lack of positive reappraisal since, I'm kind of alone on that it seems. And for the longest time I would pass it off as a 'guilty pleasure' of mine, embarrassed having brought it up only to get mocked by people for my using of it as an example of "great blockbusters of the early 90s".

In my twenties I would often refer to it as being a favourite example of mine when it comes to films that were "so bad that they were good" because I was ashamed to admit I liked what wasn't cool. In my thirties I started referring to it as an 'underrated gem' from "ages ago", but the reality was that I simply *liked it* very much. Unpretentiously and unabashedly. I liked it and I cared too much what other friends, movie geeks, etc. thought to stand behind liking it.

But then the older I got and the more I came to look at myself and my mental health differently the more I started to move towards a place of... well... being *settled* with being me and who I am.

And you know what?

With that comes the fact that I'm old enough and brave enough to find nothing 'guilty' in liking Bird on a Wire. Nor do I have to pretend it's only good because its allegedly so bad. I listen to Barry Manilow and Neil Diamond when I'm driving and not in a kitschy singalong 'take the piss' way. I listen to them because I love the compositions and the songwriting.

I would throw expensive 'posh' crisps in the bin to be able to have a couple of packets of Iced Gems instead. All these funky-flavoured IPA beers and lagers don't come close to matching an ice cold properly served pint of Heineken or a chilled bottle of Pabst Blue Ribbon...

I don't pretend otherwise anymore. And I like that about myself.

Bird on a Wire is *good* because it is pure confection with another terrific Hans Zimmer score and pleasing chemistry between Mel Gibson and Goldie Hawn (the former only stepping in to replace the latter's real-life long term boyfriend, Kurt Russell, because he was still stuck on the troubled production that was Tango & Cash!) and sometimes you just want a film that entertains you and asks nothing of you in return. This is that film.

And frankly, when I want a film that has Mel Gibson chased around the world's most improbable zoo by Kill Bill's Bill, Mac from Predator and Ned Ryerson out of Groundhog Day whilst Goldie Hawn runs away from aggressive baboons this is the ***best*** film out of all the ones where Mel Gibson is chased around the world's most improbable zoo by Kill Bill's Bill, Mac from Predator and Ned Ryerson out of Groundhog Day whilst Goldie Hawn runs away from aggressive baboons!

Like what pleases you (as long as it's legal) and embrace the pleasing feeling it gives you. You'll be amazed how much your life alters for the better when you accept doing this as the new standard and 'wear it' as a badge of honour.

There was something I found very revealing when speaking to friends and polling opinions for this book.

I asked what the one thing people were pleased to lose from their lives or let go of the moment they stopped putting too much value on 'social pressure'.

One of the predominant things I heard was "the going out".

I couldn't agree more.

There's this strong belief that 'getting old', marrying, having a family, etc. all represents this "loss of youth", and we mourn the 'death' of Saturday night pub crawls / clubbing etc. When I met my wife and the evolution occurred from 'dating' to 'co-habiting', I rejoiced in a Saturday night having grown into snuggling together on a sofa, chatting shit, watching a film, cooking or ordering a takeaway in rather than...

deep sigh

.... getting shaved and showered, ironing one of the 'good' shirts, getting out the 'going out' jeans, polishing the 'smart shoes', hitting the local pub early evening to get something to 'line the stomach', having as many pints as could be fitted in there before you got into town and the bars' there 'had your eye out' with the cost of drinks...

... squeezing into a taxi and paying double the rate, queuing to get into bars then once inside queuing to get to the bar itself, buying a round, shouting "HOW MUCH?" then shaking your head and paying anyway, drinking your drink with your elbows pushed into your shoulders whilst you get half of it nudged onto the floor by people around you...

... clocking someone you like, making eye contact with them and smiling, them smiling back, you spending so long thinking what your opening gambit with them is going to be, talking yourself out of approaching because they're far too good-looking for you and what would they see in you anyway you tell yourself and, oh look, you're mate's gone over and 'pulled' her whilst you were mentally beating yourself up...

Repeat again and again throughout the night, hit the early hours, decide that you're going to leave the club 'early' to beat the crowds at the kebab shop down the road only to get outside and realise five hundred people have all had the same thought, get your grub eventually, queue for your taxi, promise the driver you won't eat your kebab in his car but secretly sneak slithers of donner whilst he's looking the other way at junctions...

... come in, grab some drinks from the fridge, queue up a film and fall asleep in front of it then wake up late Sunday morning, look at how much you blew on a night out you didn't enjoy and vow you won't be doing *that* again – until the next Saturday because everyone is asking you why you've not found a 'nice' [woman / man] and "settled down", and you've convinced yourself the 'partner' of your dreams is going to be leant up against a pillar at quarter past one in the morning in 'Idolz Nite Klub' next to a yellowing poster that says Gareth Gates will be appearing here at 10pm... five years previously!

It's a silly token example but the fact is it can be representative of what we can do to help ourselves by looking inwards, affirming what it is that brings us positivity and what is weighing us down and *adjusting*.

Our mental health is continually fuelled by all that stuff affecting us negatively. The adjustments – choosing what we spend our money on, who we spend our time with, goals we want to work towards, jobs we no longer want to do or careers we don't wish to be a part of anymore – are all steps that put distance between where you were (in the negative) to where you want to be (in the positive) and has you outrunning your ol' black cloud with far more stamina than you probably never realised you had.

You change one thing and feel better.

Then another. And feel even more improved.

The biggest problem I faced with my mental health was the perpetual cycle:

I had episodes of depression, I took the pills, I did the therapy, I wasn't 'cured', I put this down to another example of what a failure I was and my depression worsened then I took different pills and did more intensive therapy and I still wasn't 'cured' and round and round it goes. Then I started to look inwards at my absence of self-esteem and how my value system is entirely tied to what others thought of me and I realised that therefore meant other people had far greater control over my mental health then I did myself. I didn't know much then, but I knew I didn't want that to be the case.

I decided to make two changes at the same time – the first was that I was going to reduce interactions with people who made me feel bad about myself and the second was that I was going to do something I enjoy simply because I enjoy the act of doing it. In the latter case it led to me writing three novels.

I then put a little note to myself on my phone and set an alert so that it came through as a reminder / notification every four hours. It simply said:

'You don't have to like yourself. You just have to cut yourself a little slack.'

Suddenly feelings of a depressive episode were acknowledged and met with less a thought of "Here we go again!" and more and more frequently instead a feeling of "I don't want to feel like this. What am I going to *do* about it?"

I started to see some good come from wearing the wounds of my so-called self-surgery with pride or a sense of accomplishment from how far I've brought myself mentally and emotionally.

Remember when I told you earlier on in this book about a particular Saturday night in the lead up to Christmas when I was a child?

Where I was locked in alone with a bad 'Ivan Drago' haircut and a lump on my head? And I ate myself sick watching certain films back-to-back on the telly?

I *celebrate* that time now.

Quite literally.

I am so far along from that moment, how my parents made me feel, how I felt at that time that now every year on the second Saturday in December I get a festive selection box in with some nice food and some of my favourite beer and I watch Flash Gordon and The Last Starfighter whilst snuggling with my sons, then when they're in bed my wife and I watch Running Scared and Escape From New York.

I make sure to take the time to look at my boys and to look at my wife, appreciate how far I've come and how much their love matters to me.

Furthermore, with age and self-inventory, experience, and reflection I have come to realise that weird or fat, loud or ginger, sporty or tall... creative, popular, lonely, quirky... whatever the *hell* you are in yourself, there's a place in this world for *all of us* – no matter how much gets presented before us that suggests to the contrary.

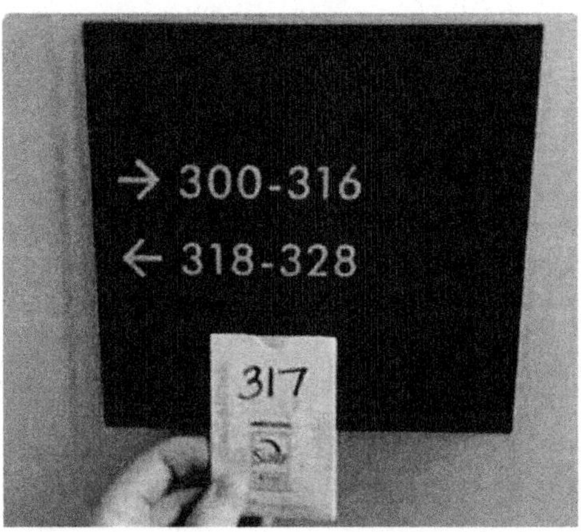

"I Feel Seen" #5

THE PRISONER OF SECOND AVENUE

I don't know how to talk about my connection to The Prisoner of Second Avenue without talking about my nervous breakdown, and I don't know how to talk about *that* without talking about my wife. I can't talk to you about my wife in relation to The Prisoner of Second Avenue without you knowing the story of 'us' so... Basically, what I'm trying to forewarn you is that I'm going to be 'going on a bit' here – way more so than probably the other chapters so if you thought *they* were a little unruly you're probably thinking "Holy fuck! How bad is this one going to be then?" whilst also inwardly questioning why I'm wasting so much time and book space on this defensive, over-explanatory 'ramble'.

In some way re-enforcing the adage that you find love when you stop looking for it, I met my wife when I went for a job interview after I had sworn off dating and relationships. I had quit a job that was making me unhappy, and I had vowed that I was going to 'work on myself'. I gave up my flat and moved in with my grandma to help take care of her because she was going through a bit of a struggle, and I looked to find a new job. I had two interviews lined up for different jobs, one permanent doing something that I wasn't entirely that interested / passionate about, but which paid a lot of money and the other a temporary job that involved working with vulnerable people.

I got offered both jobs and I was about to turn the temporary one down when my grandma interceded and stopped me from going forward with rejecting it but asking the interviewer out for a drink. "Don't follow the money," my grandma said. "Go where you could make a difference to someone's life."

I took the job and got to spend time working in the same building with this woman with the incredible smile. And we fell in love with one another (mostly whilst she taught me how to use Microsoft PowerPoint because it was integral to my job, and I didn't have any knowledge of it). This well-adjusted, middle-class optimist and the fucked-up, working class cynic.

You know, I used to mock my wife as being naïve or gullible around people because of the outlook she had towards them. Yet part of falling in love with her was realising that she treated everyone with the utmost kindness and compassion until they gave her a reason not to, whereas I entered every engagement with anyone naturally assuming I was going to be mocked, abused, taken advantage of, and stayed thinking this until I was proven wrong which I felt I rarely was.

And it was *me* who was incorrect in my approach with people through years of mistreatment. She taught me that.

We moved in together and built a life.

We got a dog and the dog turned out have this wonderful ability to spot my 'black cloud' looming and help me in ways that still kind of freak me out to this day and that I don't quite understand. Like the time I was sat on the phone to my mother, and she was saying something particularly cruel to me about how I was living my life that was quietly upsetting me when the dog sat up from being stroked and knocked the phone away from my ear and started licking the side of my head where the phone had been.

I proposed to my wife using PowerPoint.

Which is cooler than you're going to give me credit for.

Because within the slides she once taught me how to make were recordings I'd obtained from some willing celebrities and famous folk she liked, all asking her to marry me on my behalf.

[Admittedly the sheen has been taken off a couple of celeb contributions because they're now what you call "disgraced" types – all I'll say is how was I to know that one novelty 1990s pop duo were going to turn out to be such rabid anti-vaccine Covid-deniers?]

We married and had a fabulous honeymoon.

Our first child was conceived not through timed intent (although we were looking to start a family fairly immediately) but because my wife distracted me with sex to stop me from paying $24.99 on hotel pay-per-view to watch the 2014 Michael Bay produced version of Teenage Mutant Ninja Turtles at 0325 in the morning whilst suffering from *killer* jetlag.

I nearly lost her in childbirth and I can still taste the panic-induced sickness in the back of my throat to this very day from the moment when my swaddled first born son was put in front of me, and we were left in the corner of the room together whilst my wife was wheeled away from me "to surgery urgently" without anyone explaining to me what the surgery was for, how serious it was or when she would be back.

I kept asking and each uniformed medical person said someone "would be along in a moment" to explain. For the longest time no one came and my wife's final words to me as she was wheeled from the room ("Take care of our son for me!") were starting to feel way too foreboding.

I sat rocking my son whilst gently singing Tom Petty's 'Walls' to him ("... 'Cause you got a heart so big it could crush this town. And I can't hold out forever. Even walls fall down. And all around your island there's a barricade. It keeps out the danger. It holds in the pain. Sometimes you're happy. Sometimes you cry. Half of me is ocean. Half of me is sky...") because I couldn't think of any nursery rhymes off the top of my head, there and then in that moment. And that song – as well as There Might Be Giant's 'Birdhouse In Your Soul' – are the only ones I can routinely remember the words to.

I remember how I kept looking round the birthing suite at the blood-drenched floor and wishing I'd done better at GCSE biology because there was part of me that thought there shouldn't be *that* much blood come out of a person and if there was how could they survive, but I didn't know for certain... and I remember thinking that I'd come to experience a life with my wife in it and I didn't ever want to go back to the version where she wasn't there - because that version was shit.

Then, right in the middle of that thought, a nurse came and got me and my baby boy and led us to a cubicle where my wife was lying, and she got to hold him properly for the first time. Her first words to me seemed to be oblivious to my tear-filled eyes as she said "They offered me toast but then haven't brought any. Can you chase that up for me because I'm starving!"

My wife's difficult childbirth took a long time to recover from. In the ten months and change that followed the arrival of my beautiful baby son, I came to experience a feeling of love for my child I had never experienced before inside of myself but with it this constant feeling that I was not good enough to deserve this human being and that he deserved better than me as a 'guiding light' in his life.

This was aligned with all the sleeplessness that comes with a new-born, some devastating personal issues my wife and I had to deal with and which drained us mentally at a time when we weren't exactly overflowing with mental fortitude anyway, the worsening health of her grandfather whilst I was quietly having to address a [later affirmed] feeling my own beloved grandmother was in a much worse state of health than she was letting on, financial strain, the death of our adored family dog who had been a massively therapeutic 'crutch' to me and... and...

To this day I cannot explain it any other way than to say that a switch inside of me got turned off.

One minute I was arguing with my wife and her father about the tsnumai of awfulness we were trying unsuccessfully to manage, and the next *months* had passed, and I was just starting to 'wake up'.

I'm not kidding. I hadn't been in a coma or anything like that. I'd simply broken down once and for all.

I apparently slumped down into the chair in the corner of our living room that night and... *stopped.*

All my recollections after that are fitful flashes of moments that on recovery, I had my wife affirm as 'truth' or 'imaginary'.

I would come to learn that I had a nervous breakdown and that upon my wife calling the Mental Health Crisis Team for advice a trio of professionals trooped into my home the next morning, assessed me as not being a risk to myself or others thus not needing to be sectioned and prescribed me a dose of diazepam that ostensibly 'ended my days' whilst waiting for a mental health therapist to become available for me to see.

When I say 'ended my days', that's no excessive dramatic flourish.

When it comes to mental health, i.e. anxiety, for example the recommended dosage for diazepam is starting at 2mg three times a day and this can be increased to between 5mg and 10mg.

The Crisis Team started me out on 15mg, twice a day.

Then after a week they apparently realised that this was "wrong", so it became 10mg three times a day – leaving me sat comatose and unable to speak properly or co-ordinate my body, which is a crushing side effect to have when you want to be able to hold your baby son.

I'm told my wife dragged me in - literally hoisted me with her arms under my armpits to walk me like a puppet because my legs weren't that great on their own – to our GP who was aghast at the medication I'd apparently been prescribed and altered it accordingly.

I finally got put in front of my assigned psychotherapist and... remember me telling you about the one who spent our time together showing me bikini-clad holiday photos of herself on her phone whilst recommending the location of where she'd just come back from? Yup. That was *her*!

I didn't think I'd ever love my wife more than the days she gave me my children. But the more the chemical-controlled 'fug' lifted and the more I started to gain back control over my life.

And the more that happened the more I started to recognise that my wife was essentially some form of super-human:

She was raising a new-born son whilst in ill-health herself, looking after me, running a home, engaging with mental health services, challenging shitty aspects of said services, keeping us financially above water, worrying about her own father's well-being as *his* dad's condition worsened... and she never once complained or projected guilt.

I woke up in the middle of the night and found her sitting in our son's nursing chair that had, at some point during the peak of my breakdown, been moved into the corner of our bedroom near to the window. I found her asleep there and I nudged her to come back to bed.

The next morning, I spoke to her about sleeping in the nursing chair when there was no baby there to nurse and she explained to me at the worst of my overdosage on diazepam I would wake in a daze in the middle of the night and try to "get out the window", totally unaware as to where I was.

She had started to get so worried that she wasn't going to get woken by one of my attempts that she had voluntarily taken to sleeping in the chair on the route between the bed and the window so I couldn't get past her, and she'd just sort of got used to doing that.

I excused myself and overcome with a feeling of guilt that she'd felt she had to do that and awash in this sudden rush of an emotion akin to falling in love with her all over again, I went into the toilet and cried.

On the road back out of the most impactive mental episode of my life, I came across Melvin Frank's 1975 film version of Neil Simon's 1971 Broadway play, The Prisoner of Second Avenue.

If ever there was a film I should *not* have been exposing myself to whilst in recovery from a nervous breakdown it was the story of a man who suddenly loses his job and suffers a nervous breakdown which forces his wife to adapt to the new devastating reality of their lives, whilst the city around them endures an intense summer heat wave, a prolonged garbage strike and an increase in crime which they themselves fall foul to at the worst possible time.

The problem was I got 'hooked' on an exchange between Mel (Jack Lemmon) and his wife Edna (Anne Bancroft) that was almost verbatim a conversation my wife and I had conducted with one another within the peaks and troughs of my own breakdown:

Edna: *"Come on, Mel. I haven't seen you since breakfast yesterday, and I'm gonna' be fast asleep in 15 minutes. Talk to me. What did you do today?"*

Mel: *"I took a walk!"*

Edna: *"Good. Where?"*

Mel: *"From the bedroom into the living room."*

Edna: *"That's all?"*

Mel: *"Mm-hmm. Then I walked back into the bedroom... and once I went into the kitchen for a glass of water. I'd say that was my high peak of the day."*

There was *something* at play here.

There was an inescapable truth.

Expectedly so as I would later learn Neil Simon based his play on his wife's uncle, who set up his own small-town newspaper only for it to fail, go bankrupt and induce a nervous breakdown, which he was helped to recover from through the love and support of his wife and her family.

Lines like "I don't know either where I am or who I am. I'm disappearing, Edna. I don't need an analyst. I need Lost & Found!" helped me feel less alone and articulate things that I had not been able to express up until that point.

I leant into the film rather than recoil from it.

Inarguably helped by the magnificent performances from Lemmon and Bancroft. There was so much of my life and my [then] struggles present and correct here on screen.

It certainly helped that it is a *very* funny film with some tremendous dialogue ("Maybe it's not even a nervous breakdown. Doctors can be wrong, too. They took out all my top teeth... then found out it was kidney stones!" or the scene when Edna reaches out to Mel's brother Harry for help as her husband crumbles: "I thought you wanted to do something, help him." "We do want to help him!" "Then help him!" "Not when he's sick. When he's better, we'll help him.").

The Prisoner of Second Avenue didn't just make me feel *seen*, it made me look at my wife differently and develop an even greater appreciation for her than I had already.

I saw so much of what Bancroft's Edna said and did in things my wife had said and done too – all with a baby never more than one metre from her person, all on little to no sleep and all with the trials and tribulations of the day within her own life to deal with.

'Edna Edison':
"I have no strength left. Nothing. I couldn't even open my pocketbook on the bus today. A little boy had to help me."

'Mel Edison':
"You have strength, Edna!"

'Edna Edison':
"I have ***anger****! No strength!"*

The better I felt from coming out the other side of my nervous breakdown the clearer an understanding of my mental health I gained and what I needed to do and avoid doing to help improve it and take control of it.

Like with Lemmon's character in this film though, most of my strength was drawn from my wife and I had to make sure that I didn't weaken her in the process.

That she never did, or at least ever allow me to see her weaken, was one of the most staggeringly impressive displays of human resilience and strength I have encountered in my own life so far.

She was fiercely protective of me throughout what I endured in a way and on a level I had not had another person do for me.

Ever.

Getting better for her and the family we were building together, being respectful as to the courage she was displaying and the sacrifices she was making was more impactive on my overcoming a nervous breakdown than any one tablet or minute of therapy.

Your Mould Spores

I was 37 years of age when my grandma died after fighting the final strands of a terminal illness that she admitted to me in her final days she had hid from the family for “quite some time”, after I told her I had suspicions she had been poorly for a lot longer than she had made out. She dealt with her final days with such good humour and dignity. When she died, I can say I have quite honestly never felt an emotional pain like it.

The woman was a legend, not just to me but to people locally and to every one of my girlfriends and friends who met her.

My wife frankly adored her, and she was right to as well.

My grandma suffered from malapropisms and as a result once told me she thought my driving was "too erotic". (She meant “erratic” just in case you didn’t pick up on that!) When I was 10 years of age, she took on an escaped goat with my school bag (seriously!) to stop it from charging me and when it came back for another go she slapped it in the face.

Yes, you read that right.

She seemed to have a weird addiction to letting fat people know they were fat. She loved to dance and lived to sing – sometimes she did it alone in her living room with the blinds open simply because she wanted to, and she didn’t care.

When I struggled to make friends, she would pick up a bat and ball, take me out onto the field in front of her house and play the games I would play if I had had them.

She lived her life in the daily belief that, quote unquote, [hers] can't be that bad because [she's] never been on Jeremy Kyle" (back when The Jeremy Kyle Show was a thing!).

She once sat on a bus for nine hours to come to London and bring me black grapes when I'd been stabbed – a trip my own parents declined to accompany her on because it clashed with a football game they had tickets for.

There's no two ways about it, she saved me from alcoholism.

There was a period in my life where I gave up my flat and moved in with her to look after her because she was struggling with some things at that point in her life.

Whilst living together she once walked in on me having sex with a woman I'd snuck into the house whilst I thought she was out on a day trip and her only words were "Either I'm out of touch or you two are doing it wrong!"

My grandad once came home and found her walking around with paint cans tied to her feet and me pretending to stab her with a letter-opener and she explained that she was pretending "to be the giant from The Princess Bride", only for him to simply sigh and take his newspaper into the back room without asking any follow-up questions.

She was the first up to dance at my wedding at the age of (then) 91 and kept dancing alone without a fuck given until others got up and joined her. She loved a specific table overlooking the sea at a pub down the coast.

And... best of all.... she was not just my partner-in-crime for 37 years; she was my best friend and in a lot of ways my entire actual family rolled into one.

We were close from the moment I was born and as far as I'm concerned her and my grandfather as good as 'adopted' me from the time I was 12.

We had been inseparable ever since, talking on the phone at least every other day (even when I was living overseas) and going for lunch once a week when I was living back in my hometown.

The only truly consistent compliment I ever routinely received was how old fashioned I am in my manners.

That was *ALL* down to my grandma who said hello to everyone on the street regardless of if she knew them, told me from the youngest of ages "You smile at every person until they give you a reason not to!" and demanded I never walk through a door ahead of a female.

My final days spent with my grandma were ruined by the behaviour of my parents and my sister as they rushed to marshal a 'crisis' and made decisions about her final days contrary to her wishes, and which I still carry the guilt of not being able to properly challenge at that time because my mental health was in freefall.

We still managed to find time to sit and talk just like we did in her living room over the years, only this time the conversation had a finality to it that was killing me internally. She talked about how she felt she had pushed me to maintain a relationship with my parents for *her* sake because she couldn't be bothered with the hassle from my father otherwise. She told me that there was "no more that [I] can do there" and that I must "do what's right by [my] own family now".

She joked that she'd made peace with the fact her funeral was going to be full of songs she didn't want and that my brother-in-law would be a pallbearer when she couldn't stand him, because my sister had taken charge of the arrangements. "She's been arranging my funeral for the last twenty years, has that lass." She laughed before adding that she didn't care and that part of getting old was learning what was worth caring about, and how stuff like that certainly wasn't worth it.

I didn't talk about how I knew she'd been dying for a lot longer than was now being formally presented nor the impact this had on my mental health in the preceding six to eight months.

Even when she brought up the fact that she knew herself but didn't go to a doctor because they'd start talking about "treatments" and she "couldn't be bothered with all that" and, most agonisingly of all, she didn't want to tell my parents about some of her ailments in the last year because she worried my sister would drive them to put her into a residential care home.

In a quiet moment she gripped my hand and said she didn't feel like she could go because she was worried about me. I asked her why she was worried, and she said, "Because you keep trying to please people that can't be pleased rather than pleasing yourself."

I told her she didn't have to worry about me, and I squeezed her hand.

My final words to her were to thank her for never giving up on me in my life when everyone else seemed to. She replied, "You never give me a reason to!" and I bawled all the way home, telling myself that I'd finally made peace with the fact she was going to go that night.

And she did.

The minute she died I suddenly felt less safe in this world because she wasn't in it.

I got the call from my parents in the early hours of the morning and drove down to the hospice to see her one final time.

I sat down next to her lifeless body, surrounded by my parents and my sister as they talked about the funeral arrangements within the first hour of my grandma having died and I quietly looked to each of them whilst thinking over and over again about what my grandma had said to me less than ten hours earlier:

"You keep trying to please people that can't be pleased."

I left the hospice and drove to my grandma's house, letting myself in with my key and sitting down on the living room right in front of the fireplace I'd spent my childhood, watching video tapes, eating her food, and snuggling myself into her sheepskin rug.

I closed my eyes, and I could see William Phelps' 1987 underdog surfer movie North Shore playing in the corner of the room with my grandma coming in, tutting and saying "You've not put this on again have you?"

I could see the much-maligned Cannon & Ball film The Boys In Blue, with my grandma and grandad laughing uproariously at Bobby Ball.

And Tough Enough too – the 1983 drama about a country-and-western singer (Dennis Quaid) who enters a fighting tournament to pay his family's bills and who must choose between his accidental success as a brawler and his ambitions as a musician.

Yes, that is a *real* film that *really* exists.

One which my grandma in particular seemed to have a soft spot for – but not as much of a soft spot as the one she had for the musical TV movie My Boyfriend's Back, with the lady from LA Law teaming up with the star of Who's The Boss I had a weird crush on (Judith Light!) and the woman from that hit sitcom I always forget the name of (Google tells me it was Sandy Duncan and the show was The Hogan Family, and I can't *believe* I would forget her seeing as she starred in Disney's The Cat From Outer Space), and they played estranged members of ex-60s group getting back together in middle-age for a live TV concert.

I thought back to that time when I was 8 years and my parents did their atypical 'school holiday' tactic of driving me to my grandparents, stopping at the local video rental shop on the way, renting a couple of tapes of whatever family films were available on the £1 (non-premium) shelf and then dumping me there until they'd finished work / come back from a day out, etc. And I *loved* when they did it.

That's how I first experienced Pee Wee's Big Adventure and it's no exaggeration to say I'd never seen anything or anyone in Paul Reubens' Pee Wee Herman like that before. It absolutely dropped my jaw. I loved it. (I still do!) It made me laugh so hard. Of course, my grandparents HATED it. But I *lived* for it and kept pushing for it to get rented again and again.

I sat alone in the dark of that living room and I cried.

I smiled a little bit too.

I then exited to go upstairs and say goodbye to the spare back bedroom that held many happy memories of sleepovers and to take away a photo of my grandma and I from her chest of drawers that I knew she kept there.

It was one of my favourites.

My jaw dropped when I went upstairs and found that the entire bedroom had already been boxed up, drawers emptied, pictures taken down, you name it.

Someone had been in here packing up her belongings before she'd even died. I was sickened.

I looked down at one of the bin-liners and noticed a 'doodle' that was familiar. I picked it up and saw that it was a drawing I had done as a child. Underneath it was more drawings I had scribbled.

Underneath them was silly stories I had written at a young age and comic strips I had created that I had no memory of ever having done.

There was a copy of my A-level film studies essay on Clint Eastwood's Unforgiven that I'd scored so well in writing that the examining board kept it as a 'test example'.

Everything I had ever created. And I mean ever.

Every doodle, every scrap of paper, every silly story... my grandma had kept the lot, and it was all scrunched up and tipped into a bin liner ready to be chucked.

She had kept everything, and my family's response was not to have put it together for me to look through and consider keeping anything or to give it a mere seconds thought – they took it from wherever it was my grandma had been keeping it all and they tipped it straight into a bin bag.

I broke down sobbing in a way I had never done before and have never cried like since.

I was in absolute *agony*.

I cuddled the bin liner full of paper like I was cuddling my grandma herself and then, finally, I composed myself to leave.

And whilst sat in my car down the street from her front door, drying my eyes and getting ready to drive home, I saw my sister drive into the street.

She didn't see me parked a little further up, but she alighted and removed empty boxes and bags, heading into my grandma's house to 'finish the job'. It was ten to six in the morning.

She could have gone home to rest or get breakfast ready for her children who would be waking soon. No, *this* was my sister's priority. My grandma had been dead less than a couple of hours.

Something broke in me that day, especially with regards to my family. I couldn't articulate it then any more than I can properly now but their conduct in the final days of my grandma's life drove home that I didn't just have any respect for them, I had no actual affection for them either.

I didn't *like* them.

Why then had I spent so much of my life trying to obtain validation from them? I had to get an answer to that question, I felt.

The funeral was a daze.

I delivered a eulogy in keeping with my grandma's request to make it funny, not 'soppy'. I wore a grey suit rather than a black one because she told me I looked "better in grey than black".

After the funeral as I stood outside the plethora of mourners, reflective of how truly loved my grandma was within her community, poured out of the church and shook my hand and told me what they thought of my eulogy.

I looked across at my dad and saw him seething.

My sister glared at me, whispered in his ear and he nodded in agreement with whatever she had said.

I looked at my sister and I was reminded of something my grandma said a few months before her death about my parents handing "complete control of the family" over to my sister as a teenager and "we've all been the worse for it since".

Once talking to my wife, my grandma described my parents' relationship with my sister as "a sickness [her] and [my] grandad never understood".

I don't know why it hit me right there and then in that moment outside the church, but it did – I realised I *hated* my family.

My wife and I didn't go to the wake afterwards.

Instead alongside her parents and my baby son, I had booked my grandma's favourite table overlooking the sea at that pub she liked down the coast.

We went and sat together there, had a meal, and told funny stories about my grandma, like the infamous goat fight and that time she stood in her kitchen with a cup of tea and said to me and my wife "Sue is out there showing off her fifteen thousand pound caravan. You can hear her going on about it being for the weekends when her and her partner go 'roughing it'! But one, you can't call it 'roughing it' when you're staying in a £15,000 caravan and two, she can't call him her 'partner' when he's married to someone else and only sees her at the weekend – which is what I think the caravan is for!" And suddenly, this voice shouted through the open kitchen window "I can hear you; you know!" and my grandma replied "Sorry Sue! Just gossiping, pay no mind!"

In the months that followed I made no effort with my parents, partly because the 'tissue' that connected us was gone but mainly because I was starting to process some pretty huge feelings:

I *hated* my family, I *hated* how they had raised me, I *hated* the outlook in life they'd projected onto me, I *hated* the abuse both emotionally and physically that had been bestowed upon me and I *hated* how they made me feel when I was around them.

So why had I spent so long chasing their respect or their approval?

I came to realise that it had <u>nothing</u> to do with them as people.

It had zero to do with me wanting their respect because of who they were as individuals.

The best that could be surmised was that I chased it because I just assumed that because they were my family I was *meant* to have their affection and their esteem.

I did it because I looked at other people and their relationship with their family and I thought I should have that too; that there was something wrong with me because my family withheld it.

I wasn't sleeping. I wasn't eating well. I had a baby, and my wife was still in recovery from a complicated childbirth. I missed my grandma terribly.

Then in the early hours of one morning I went upstairs and found my wife breastfeeding in the nursing chair tucked in the dark corner of my son's nursery.

I quietly approached her and whispered "I always felt there was something wrong with me because of the love and the respect my family withheld from me, especially comparative to my sister. But you know what? There was something wrong with *them*!"

The next day I attended a therapy appointment and talked through my feelings with the counsellor. I said that there was part of me that knew I needed to 'cut the cord' between myself and my family but that in doing so I would have 'no one'.

The counsellor replied "You have your wife and your new son. You have your in-laws, who I've seen you speak with more warmth about than you have your blood family."

She then set me a challenge there and then – to tell her *one* happy memory from my childhood involving my parents or my sister.

I talked about those Sunday afternoons with my grandparents.

I talked about the summer spent making 'movies' with my then best friend and our trips all over to watch the sort of films we'd never normally get a chance to see on our doorstep.

I talked about all these little random things and moments, and each time the counsellor gently reminded me that none of them – not a single one – featured my parents or was driven by my parents' involvement.

"The best you can muster," she said, "is the Saturday nights they would go out and you were left from a young age watching films and eating popcorn and that's because you were alone, and they were not there to hurt or upset you. That is quite revealing."

My wife and I went for a walk with our son later that day, and I talked through where my head was at:

What sort of relationship are my parents going to be able to forge with our son or any of our other children down the line, I asked.

It's not like they're going to be called on to babysit like traditional grandparents would because after what they did to me growing up, I don't trust them to be alone with my kid(s).

It's not like we're going to go for dinner dates with my sister and her wet blanket husband because we find many of their world views to be abhorrent and self-centred.

So, what *would* this familial relationship look like going forward?

"I've never said this out loud before," I said to my wife. "But I've served my country, I've travelled to the other side of the world, I've got up and tried stand-up comedy, I've boxed, and I've always tried to do my best in life... I've done vastly more with my life so far than all of them combined yet when I'm in their company I shrink. I fucking *shrink*. And I hate how I feel about myself around them and I hate that I let them have this power."

I decided right there and then that they were not going to have that power or control over how I feel about myself anymore.

The sort of people who behaved how they did around my grandma as she died were not the sort of people I wanted in my life and wanted as influences upon my son.

There's this terrific Frightened Rabbit song, 'Break in the Clouds', that goes:

"I've been sitting on a feeling, trying to figure it out. It's difficult to see through those clouds." and "Hold on, hold on. You're not done yet. Hold on, hold on. The sun has not set."

The song goes on to indicate that we don't give up, but we don't sit and wait for a 'break in the clouds' either. We get proactive with the feeling.

So, I did.

With my parents removed from my life via a letter I sent to them explaining I no longer wanted a relationship with them, I started to look at who I was exactly – but more specifically who I wanted to be going forward at 38 years of age.

It wasn't overnight or instant.

It wasn't easy and it took some getting used to challenging thoughts and holding them to evidential account.

I held myself to task for not fighting for my grandma in her final days as hard as I should have in the face of my family's behaviour as well as the choices my dad made hiding behind being the "next of kin".

I felt embarrassment and guilt that I did not do for her what she would have done for me, after thirty-plus years of fighting my corner when no one else would.

I realised that the singular reason I did was not out of any deference to my family. It was because I was in a poor state mentally at the time and didn't have the strength.

I was deeply ashamed of that. I still am in many ways.

I decided I was not going to ever allow the so-called 'black cloud' to have such a control over me again that I was not able to protect those that I loved.

I vowed to get to work - on myself.

I started to realise that I wasn't a bad person at all.

I'd told myself I was because of how people treated me.

I must be *this* because I'm treated like *that*, you know?

The reality was that I am not a cruel man or a selfish one. I don't maliciously hurt nor subjugate other people. I could hurt peoples' feelings without intending to through clumsy choices of words or a lack of sensitivity in a situation where sensitivity was imperative.

But I have a big heart that's driven by a desire to treat everyone how I want to be treated myself, and I was all too quick to harbour emotional distress when this wasn't reciprocated.

I am too eager, and I talk too much because I am frequently nervous and uncomfortable around people, and I mask that by filling silences or by displaying fake confidence.

I am prone to driving people away because of this.

Yet am I deserved of being bullied because of this element of who I am? Is it strong enough justification to mock and belittle me?

No.

I had reached a stage of personal strength where I didn't know that I was merited for much, but I knew that this sort of behaviour was unearned and that was a good enough start. I had lived a [frequently mocked] 'varied' life, sure. And with that came various experience in a multitude of different things. With experience comes knowledge, and with knowledge comes a greater understanding.

I had *something* to offer.

For the first time in 38 years, I realised that I genuinely had something to offer.

We looked at exercise earlier on and it's interesting that in that specific area we are willing to accept that if we turn up or step out to exercise and we do the *same* amount of reps for the *same* amount of sets with the *same* amount of weights, or we run the exact *same* distance for the exact *same* amount of time with no variable change whatsoever over and over again over time we will not progress.

Our body simply becomes accustomed to the standard. But we seem resistant to accepting this in all facets of our life, especially our mental health.

I know that I did myself for the longest time:

Just do whatever it is my parents want, just do whatever my colleagues want of me, just do whatever this friend wants to do because that will make them happy and if they're happy they'll like me and if they like me I'll feel validated, and that will make me feel good about myself and that I have worth.

Time and again I followed this process and time and again it yielded no positive outcome and affected me negatively in terms of my mental health, each episode of depression or anxiety reinforcing the idea that I was a failure.

I changed nothing but expected change regardless.

We have a bizarre tendency to do the same thing over and over with no variable change and expect different results and then complain about our status quo.

I never really 'got' something my grandad used to say to me when I was growing up until much, much later in my life but one of his favourite analogies was this:

"If every day you got up to leave the house and every time you opened your front door there was a big muscley fella waiting on the doorstep and he kicked you square in the nuts, how often would you keep opening the door or how quickly would you convince yourself to just stop trying to leave the house before you eventually got round to thinking 'Hey, I might try going out through the back door'?"

With the removal of my family from my life came the decision to proactively work on my self-esteem and my confidence.

With that came the unavoidable task of taking a closer look at my mental health and my relationship to it; the very idea that issues of depression / anxiety and so forth didn't keep returning because I couldn't 'beat' them - they just never actually left.

They were *always there*, part of who I am and part of my life experience and outlook, and they simply needed to be treated in a way that let them know I was in control of them and not the other way around.

You can get all sorts of sprays and treatments to remedy a mould problem in your home. The mould sometimes comes back, and needs treated again.

It doesn't mean that you didn't clean the mould away properly the first time, necessarily. It means that with mould spores *always being present* in our home, they will return when conditions (high humidity, for example) are favourable.

The impacted areas of our mental health are our 'mould spores'.

The negative mental health 'spores' return when conditions – work stress, money worries, loneliness, sleeplessness – are favourable.

The treatment we use on them can determine how long they go away for or how intensely they come back.

What I started to do the more I worked on my self-esteem was look at what kept the 'mould' away the longest and what proved the most impactful. The contents of this book make up what I came to realise worked for me and I hope may work for you too.

I *know* they work because I am still alive.

And because one day I heard the Distant Cousins song, 'Are You Ready', and I took it as my personal anthem:

> *"Today I take my own advice and make the most of it.*
> *Too many times my choices have been guided by my fears.*
> *Into the dark and unknown water, I will sink or swim.*
> *Like a blade of grass reaching for the sun, I'm ready to begin.*
> *I keep on climbing, up against the wind..."*

Embracing The Small Stuff: Finding Joy

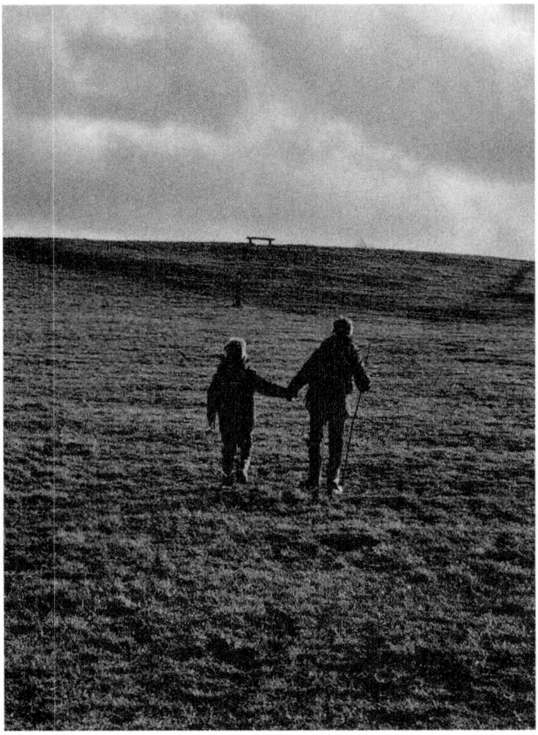

I know I touched on it earlier, but I must reiterate again how fascinating you start to see certain facets and factors in your life when you're looking at them as positive or negative fuel towards your mental and emotional wellbeing. The more in control you become of your mental health...

… certainly when you're taking the time to self-reflect, set yourself goals, push yourself to exercise a little, hold yourself to account, etc…
the more you genuinely start to question why you willingly expose yourself to things that affect you adversely.

It's undoing your hard work.

The same goes with the things that *help* with your emotional state.

I grew up being mocked and beaten for enjoying writing and watching films and so the notion that I could draw positive developments in my mental health by leaning into those very things that I was chastised and punished for throughout my teenage years and my adolescence?

That took a *long* time to get my head around and embrace.

Then one day I started writing – not for a job or with deadlines, or with any goal in mind. I just started writing as a hobby of sorts and I enjoyed it. I found a keyboard and a blank page intoxicating and the flow of words to be bizarrely relaxing.

I wrote a couple of journals, some of which came to form the spine of this book. I opened a Letterboxd account and started posting film reviews, making some lovely friends within that community along the way.

I even wrote a trilogy of fictional private eye thrillers that I published, which *appear* to have been well-received and enjoyed by those that have read them.

And I started asking friends and others who have suffered with depression, trauma, stress or mental health issues the same question:

Do you lean in on the things that make you happy when you're having a bad day, or do you push yourself to do the things others recommend for you instead / the things you *think* you should be doing as opposed to the things you *want* to do?

I was legitimately shocked to find that so many don't do the former, that they dismiss those enjoyable or pleasurable things as 'silly' or something they are not wanting to risk being tainted by a "bad mood".

One friend told me she now knits because when she had anxiety issues growing up her aunty used to knit with her and she found it helped her as a child, so she took it back up in adulthood, finding it to be very therapeutic.

Another friend hilariously wrote back to me and said:

"Mate, I'm not the person to speak to on this. I still take hot baths and light candles after a horrendous day and a low mood because I'm repeatedly told how relaxing it can be. I hate baths and I spend the whole time thinking I'm going to burn the house down and end up getting out more stressed than when I went in. And yet time and again I run a bath and light a candle."

We often formulate what is 'good' for our mental state around what we *think* we should be doing, what our friends are telling us to do or what counsellors are suggesting we 'take up'.

The reality is that our emotional state improves positively when we do things that we like and enjoy, not when we do the things that we presume will make a friend or family member happy.

I had that problem with one particular friend in my life that I sadly had to end a friendship with because they were routinely telling me what would "make [me] better" and that I just needed to come out with them on these "crazy" nights out and "drink through it", and I knew that this wasn't what was good for me mentally or financially at that time.

Especially when I was trying to evaluate my negative relationship with alcohol.

On they pushed with this angle and the guilt that they would project onto me if I chose not to go out or do what they wanted "for me". If a friend is telling you that what is in your best interests is *their* best interests, they're not a friend.

There's a special place at the bottom of the totem pole for folk who spot lonely people desperate for friendship and manipulate that for their own gain.

The greatest suggestion I can make to you when it comes to 'feeding' your mental health properly is to 'design' your perfect day.

Where would you go?

What would you do?

Who would you be with?

Would something have to happen for so-called perfection to *occur* or would those first three elements coming together be sufficient in themselves?

I did this again and again as an 'exercise' at both ends of my mental health journey and you know what? It was always such bullshit.

I repeatedly lied to myself about what I should be doing or that I needed to go somewhere that I'd not been before or nonsense like that, and... and... so much of it was filled with things that I knew *other people* would enjoy and perhaps I would get enjoyment from by proxy.

It was all pub crawls or weekends away, sometimes it was receiving the promotion I was deserved of at work and then going out for a meal to celebrate – like my perfect state of happiness was tied to validation at work.

One time I even wrote about going to Glastonbury.

Like what the *fuck*?

Anyone who knows me knows how laughable that is. I mean, my wife took me to see Bon Jovi as a surprise when we were first dating and midway through the concert she asked if I was enjoying myself (because it has been said I mainly have a resting 'not having fun' face!) and I replied "Yes, but it would be even better if all these other people weren't here!"

I couldn't even be honest with myself about what my perfect day was. Then one day it *happened*. The perfect day itself. Not me writing out what it would look like.

It was a couple of years back, on a Sunday.

And it happened by accident.

My wife and my sons, along with my in-laws, headed out for a morning walk around an old country park next to where I grew up, a place I spent so much of my childhood on my bike.

The sky was overcast, there was a coldness in the air and we were all wrapped up as my youngest boy jumped in every puddle he could find whilst my eldest walked alongside me holding my hand and I pointed out places and things around the country park from when I was a boy:

"... Over there was where I built this 'base' out of branches and leaves and hung out in it all day reading comics, this was where I used to ride my bike to the top of and then speed down back when it was all gravel and not flowers like it is now, and over there was where we used to go sledging on the rare winters when it snowed heavily enough and one time I hit a rock so hard on the way down it snapped my plastic sledge clean in half..."

... Then the rain came and we sludged back home.

We threw our clothes straight in the wash and were in warm, dry pyjamas by early afternoon.

My youngest son played happily on the floor with toys.

My wife cooked a lamb roast dinner.

I showed my eldest son film clips of Bobcat Goldthwaite in the likes of the Police Academy sequels, Hot to Trot and One Crazy Summer and talked about how I thought he was the funniest person *ever* when I was growing up.

My eldest laughed hard at the clips (especially the Godzilla bit from One Crazy Summer) and that got us talking about Pee Wee Herman, which in turn led to watching Pee Wee's Big Adventure for the first time together with a blanket over us.

Pee Wee's Big Adventure is so intrinsically its own thing, so unashamedly comfortable in being silly and fun. There is everything at play there that should never, *ever* work... and yet it does – effortlessly.

It is a 'character' piece in which the main character is as beloved to some as he is polarising to others, set within the constructs of a standard 'road' movie, and executed like a live action cartoon. It should be an utter car crash.

And yet it is a masterpiece.

Watching it with my eldest, he initially looked at me like I was mad for most of it and didn't really seem to forgive me after the infamous 'Large Marge' bit. BUT then he came round because he did love and laugh hard at the cliff fall, the "Tequila" bit and, of course "*Paging Mr. Herman. Mr. Herman you have a telephone call at the front desk!*" which nearly broke him from laughing so much.

I sat listening to my youngest son innocently and enthusiastically play on the floor and I looked at my eldest and was reminded that hearing either of my children laugh hard is one of my favourite sounds in the whole world.

My wife found some of my cherished Pabst Blue Ribbon at the back of the fridge and brought through a glass, then we sat together and ate this fabulous roast dinner as the grey sky darkened and the rain smashed down outside the window.

My youngest climbed up onto my chest and fell asleep in my arms, Pee Wee's Big Adventure ended and we put The Rocketeer on afterwards.

James Horner's gorgeous music soared, Joe Johnson's sublime on-point direction married with the [then] modern effects and decidedly old-fashioned storytelling, and those majestic action sequences played out as the Rocketeer fought Nazis... and FBI agents... and the Mafia, all in a sweet, good-natured and dryly funny 1990s masterpiece that is one of the greatest and most underappreciated comic book movies of all time...

... and I looked around this room, right there in that moment and felt like the luckiest man on the planet.

This woman saw something in me no one else did or has since and she married me and gave me these two amazing children, and these children don't love me because of my successes or my failures, or how rich or popular I am.

They love me because I love them and care for them and make them feel safe. And they make *me* feel safe.

They love me because to them I'm 'Dad'.

That's it.

That's all.

And to them that's more than enough.

I'd never been happier than I was in that moment right there and then, discovering a feeling of pure and unadulterated joy in the smallest of things; a rainy Sunday snuggled with my wife and children.

I realised that the dream would be *this*, every day... coming in from a long walk and getting cuddled up on rainy afternoons, eating good food (my wife cooks a hell of a roast!), embracing the sound of my children's laughter and watching good films.

That's the thing, isn't it?

We accept that happiness and contentment are massive boons to our mental health, and we go searching for it far and wide with our arms held open as far as we can stretch them in order to embrace this huge wave of pleasure when we find it, sometimes all too oblivious to the fact that its right there in front of us in much smaller and more manageable portions than we could have ever thought possible.

We let others or outside influences propagate this notion that we must draw joy from this, that or the other.

That we must exercise a certain way for a certain amount of time, that we must go for arduous walks to the top of tall mountains and look out over magnificent vistas, holiday in beautiful places and the like.

When in fact our joy can be found in an uninterrupted lie-in, a thoughtful gift from a friend or even a good film.

It took me far too long to realise that the size, significance, and sensation of joy is ours and ours alone. It isn't for anyone else to tell you if it is sufficient for you and your mental health.

Only *you* know that.

The friend that is telling you you'll feel better if you come out and get drunk doesn't know you better than you know yourself.

If you know that a binge-drink fuelled night-out can't compete with a night in, a large home-made hot chocolate and a couple of episodes of retro television on ITV4 (by God, the days they were doing The Rockford Files and Magnum PI back-to-back was heavenly, wasn't it?), lean in on where *you* know the joy to be.

Time and again, I would struggle around Christmas because it meant being directly in the company of my family for prolonged periods of time where alcohol flowed – and resulted in moments like that time my dad told me that my brother-in-law was the son he'd always wanted, then awkwardly realised towards the end of his sentence who he was saying this to.

I *hated* Christmas.

Christmas represented second hand presents whilst my sister got brand new things.

It epitomised getting shouted at for some infraction and sent to my room whilst the rest of the family hung out downstairs.

It was flashbacks to a memory of my grandad standing towering over me as my dad charged across the living room to hit me for some reason I can't remember, putting himself as a shield between father and son as he told my dad "You hit him. I hit you." then my dad backing off and cowardly thinking better of it.

As I got older it symbolised sitting at the edge of tables or sofas, being largely ignored by everyone but my grandma, or if I was spoken to it was to ask me loaded questions about my life so my answers could be a source of mockery or criticism.

My wife is the reverse of me.

She's my opposite in many, many ways and yet somehow, we fit together.

But there was a time when this was never more apparent than the festive season, where I played the role of Bill Murray's Frank Cross from the Christmas classic Scrooged with ease, and my wife would happily take on the role of Carol Kane's Ghost of Christmas Present:

Occasionally [verbally] beating the shit out of me and dragging me towards the 'festive cheer'. Her delight in the decorations, the Christmas markets, the lights, being with her family, thinking up thoughtful gifts for people... I'm not going to lie, it *got* to me.

By the time our children were born, and she was fully / overly committed to the Christmas rituals of cookies and carrots left out the night before, Christmas pyjamas and what not, she had me fully converted and now I *adore* Christmas.

It's my favourite time of the year.

Because of her.

She infected me.

Every Christmas Eve we go for a family walk, we finalise bits and pieces, lock in the arrangements with her parents, prep some food the night before and wrap the final round of presents (she wraps, I hand across pieces of sticky tape).

Then settle down with a drink in our hands, the Christmas tree lit up and we watch Andrew Davis' The Package every year without fail.

Which she *used to* love and look forward to but is now thoroughly bored by and mostly naps through it after a glass of mulled wine.

I sit and watch this cog-whirling, intelligent, pacy, race-against-time action thriller that will leave you in the dust if you're not giving it its due attention and I'm... *happy*.

That's my wife next to me on the sofa, there's all the presents stacked up under the tree that my kids are going to go crazy for and here's Gene Hackman...

... leading a bobby dazzler of a cast (Tommy Lee Jones, Chelcie Ross, Joanne Cassidy, John Heard, Dennis Franz, Pam Grier, Reni Santoni and Harry Lennix) in service to Davis - a director who never really got the respect he deserved for being a high end helmer of action thrillers and for making one of the greatest movies of all time in The Fugitive.

I could wax lyrical about the majesty of The Package for at least an entire chapter.

It's an unjustly forgotten political thriller with a final third that is a masterwork of precision, tension building, and wall-to-wall pay-off; the end result is a film that stands as one of the best action thrillers of the 1980s and one of the all-time great conspiracy movies, especially conspiracy-driven action thrillers set around the Christmas period...

... but I'll force myself back on point:

I think back to the Christmas Eves of my teenage years, and the dread building as to what the next day was going to bring.

I'd think back to those of my twenties too, standing in packed bars and drinking through the building dread as to what the next day was going to bring then having to deal with it hungover.

I looked for happiness in going out with friends when I didn't want to, or going round to my parents to sit in the corner listening to my sister talk for eight hours whilst my parents nodded passively at her until it was time for me to go home.

I found it instead holding hands with my wife on the sofa, eating honey-roasted peanuts, drinking Pabst Blue Ribbon and watching The Package for the umpteenth time... whilst *looking forward* to the next day!

That thing you like?

That silly routine or tradition?

That small thing?

That's *yours*.

You're allowed it. Your mental health will thank you, I promise.

Part Three

Films As 'Bandages' Part I:

Films That Can Make You Laugh (aka The Dopamine Effect)

Very early on in this book we looked at antidepressants in a bit closer detail and you'll remember – *of course* you will – how we talked about neurotransmitters like serotonin that affect your mood and how antidepressants help to get the levels right with these neurotransmitters. Alongside serotonin there's hormones like dopamine, oxytocin and endorphins that play their part in your mood and emotional state too, which antidepressants are often called in to regulate and help manage as well.

But did you know that some medical studies showed that the physical act of smiling and laughing can get the neurotransmitters and hormones flowing and releasing in such a manner that many doctors refer to laughter as one of our "natural antidepressants."

Who feels like laughing when they're at their lowest though, right?

I know all too well that feeling of being so crippled with emotional pain and weight that you genuinely can't remember the last time you smiled let alone feeling in the mood to laugh.

I remember one counsellor that I was seeking treatment from commended me on my resilience in the face of persistent knock-backs and knockdowns. She complimented my sense of humour and said that if nothing else it was important for me to maintain that because psychologically humour is an excellent coping mechanism that helps with a sense of control and perspective.

I used to get secretly frustrated by this because I often wanted to scream at her that the self-deprecation and the sarcasm or whatever was often just a 'mask' or a 'barrier'. I never really had the courage to tell her that it was all a public façade and that the minute I had closed my own front door I would frequently collapse into sobbing heaps or uncontrollably shake with the sheer exhaustion of the day. Over time my perspective changed the more my assessment of my own mental health evolved, and I started to take more control over it. A sense of humour can really help put these barriers up, sometimes *much needed* barriers, between you and adversities you're facing, like a safety net or force-field in some cases.

Accessing these "natural antidepressants" aren't going to feel that easy to do when you're looking around in your life and you're seeing debt that feels insurmountable, loneliness that never seems to go away, nightmares about past traumas that are controlling your life, the loss of a loved one that you're struggling to accept or whatever your mental health impactor may be. That's where your exposure to *external* or *third party* humour becomes important – as in not trying to do things to make yourself laugh or pushing yourself to find humour in your *own* situations or feelings, but to give yourself over to somebody else's efforts in providing the so-called 'funny'.

Several studies around depression have shown that people who are in a period of low mood or despair and have been drawn to laughter through films or television show spiked positive upticks because smiling and laughter delivers the dopamine, serotonin and endorphins responsible for making people feel happy and less stressed.

Now that's not to say that laughter alone will cure all mental health ills – and the other things we're discussing in this book (medication, counselling, goal setting, outlook adjustments) all should be allowed to play their part – but it has been known to make positive impacts in our physiological state(s) and emotional health alongside uplifting and feelgood content too, which we'll look at in a separate chapter imminently.

Watching comedy can help us shift our perspectives and sometimes lessen the weight that sits upon us because we may see our woes successfully satirised or recalibrated from someone else's perspective with a degree of lightness or insight we'd not considered before. Comedies can help us to escape and provide a safe respite from the darkness we're feeling by releasing brain chemicals that help in the fight against it, or by simply proving a distraction from thoughts that have otherwise felt unrelenting up until that point.

Also, whether watched in a crowded cinema or alone in your home they have this innate power to make you feel a little bit less alone.

What I'd like to do now is recommend to you *some* of my favourite comedies that I have always found have really helped me getting the "natural antidepressants" flowing and to make me feel a little better, sometimes at incredibly low moments. I've split them (all of which I would go to bat as being hall of famer comedies for me personally) into three categories: There's what I think are the 'classics' of the genre, films that I think are really very underrated and comedies of a sort of 'absurdist' bent which I tend to find to be my favourite type of "comfort blanket" when my depression is very heavy. ['Absurdist' is just a wanky, posh, cineaste's term. What I really mean is 'stupid' or 'daft'.]

I'm an enormous unashamed fan of **My Cousin Vinny** and would fight to the death defending it as one of the best comedies of the 1990s - and one of my all-time favourite comedies, full stop.

You can 'snark' at Joe Pesci's ill-fitting wig till the cows come home, but you'd still be left with a comedy that works hard to deliver some form of comedic uplift, whether that be through its tight zinging dialogue, the performances themselves or a visual gag here and there - at least every five minutes.

It's just a wall-to-wall gift and it works tremendously as a legit courtroom drama too (there's clearly a reason why the American Bar Association consider it the third best cinematic example of trial work and understanding of rule of law.).

I return to this film at least once a year - often as a low mood pick-me-up and it never fails to serve me well! It really is a classic!

One man's 'absurdism' is another man's 'classic' but **Airplane!** is technically both. It's a spoof on disaster movies (a subgenre of cinema that I adore in its own right) that is designed to deliver a gag of some kind – verbal, visual, clever, or silly – at a minimum rate of every sixty seconds, if not *faster*. You don't have to worry or get dismissive towards it if a joke doesn't land with you because whilst you're getting set to sneer at it, another one will race up and 'get' you good.

This Is Spinal Tap is a mockumentary (aka a fake documentary) about a heavy metal band. Don't be put off by any notion that you must like or have some interest or understanding of heavy metal music as a genre of music. You absolutely don't. It's just an incredibly well-executed ego-bursting delight with the sort of comedic set-pieces that make you laugh with their ridiculousness and help you realise it takes very clever people to make these degrees of daftness land.

Stripes (the second of Bill Murray's iconic comedy 'trilogy' with the director Ivan Reitman, with their third being the sci-fi comedy horror masterpiece that is Ghostbusters) is essentially Harold Ramis and Bill Murray's anarchic version of a Hope & Crosby "*in the army now*" style picture. It may have dated badly with its casual misogyny, but it remains a funny film that I hold dear not just because it reminds me of sleepovers at my grandparents' house where my grandmother would frequently tut and leave the room whilst my grandad would stifle laughter at John Candy mud-wrestling with bikini-clad buxom blondes, but also because the things it gets criticised for – its lack of discipline and almost scatological approach to storytelling – are the things that I like *most* about it.

Albert Brooks is one of the finest and sharpest comedy talents and he's made far too few (only a handful in fact) films as writer / director. Three of his movies – Lost In America, Defending Your Life and Modern Romance – are big, *big* favourites of mine but if you want serious laughs at a rate of knots that get the dopamine flowing you've got to go back to **Real Life**, his remarkably prescient feature directorial debut where he plays a filmmaker trying to make the first ever reality documentary involving an average American family. A film he made in 1979, no less.

The Odd Couple is one of the most delightfully simple, endlessly rewarding comedies that runs perfectly even to this day on the effortlessly magnificent trifecta of putting Walter Matthau and Jack Lemmon in an apartment as two opposites whose friendship is impacted by them suddenly having to live together, with Neil Simon's flawless and immensely quotable script between them to dig their teeth into. It's been remade, rejigged and ripped off. But it's never been bettered.

What's Up Doc? is a romantic chase comedy that holds up marvellously and has a gag-per-minute ratio that makes it deserved of Airplane! levels respect. I am a big fan of it and there's not a great deal of Barbra Streisand films that I would say that about. Everyone talks about the infamous San Francisco car chase when it comes to this film and that set piece *does* still hold up fabulously, but for me the highlight of the whole thing is the climactic courtroom sequence after that with Liam Dunn gurning and twitching away. It is a great ode to a real 'lost' type of cinematic comedy.

Somewhere between the critical / commercial / awards adoration considered disproportionate at the time, the lesser sequel, and Billy Crystal's wildly uneven output since, there's a bit of a... not quite a backlash, but certainly a dismissal of **City Slickers** these days, a film I recommended to you earlier in the book.

There shouldn't be any sort of turn against this film. It's an absolute masterpiece of its type - the studio packaged comedy picture. But it's also a film that doesn't get better with age. It's a film that gets better the more *YOU* age. The story of men in mid-life crisis attempting a modern day cattle drive is not for the 14 - 35 year old demographics. This is a film for when you're in your mid 40s, sat "taking inventory" and wondering about who you are and what your footprint is in this world. And here's this silly but warm love letter to the Western to make you feel a little less alone in your thoughts at that time. I've always had an enormous soft spot for this film but the older I've got the more it's resonated much harder with me. In time I've come to see that for what it is, what it's trying to be and what it has to say... it's actually a *perfect* little film. It remains very funny, full of both heart and lovely on point performances from its three leads. (Boy oh boy, what a hard miss Bruno Kirby is huh?)

I can imagine generationally and with transgenderism having evolved in the way it has, there'll be a contingent of folk who nowadays will simply dismiss **Tootsie** – a romantic farce about an unemployable actor who disguises himself as an unknown actress to start getting work - sight unseen just from its synopsis. But I urge you not to do that because to do so would mean to miss out on a deceptively smart, very funny, and actually really rather sweet romantic comedy. It has a lot of fun with its plot complications, and as a result, it IS *a lot* of fun to indulge in; it swipes at topics as varied as sexual identity, sexism, pontificating and self-serving actors, the entertainment industry, agents... and yet moreover it turns out to be a wonderfully emotional love story. It works on absolutely every level it touches upon, even when such things should not be normally placed near one another – who'd have thought a satirical, sexual identity farce with an extremely lovely romance running through its central core could work half as well as this does.

Steve Martin spent so long in the comedic doldrums – and thankfully I grew up on his "early funny stuff" rather than what he was putting out in the 90s – that there is very nearly an entire generation who don't realise he was (and still technically is) one of the greatest comedic minds of the modern age. He's made some of the best comedies of all time. I just accept that if you were born after 1990 and didn't watch "old movies" (i.e. movies from before you were born) you'd probably not realise that. Though I will fight a bare-chested fight with anyone who doesn't think **Bowfinger** (one of the greatest satires on the movie industry there has ever been) is a funny film.

In terms of what we're going for with hard, regular laughs and lovely feelings from the release of serotonin and dopamine, etc. additional to Bowfinger, then you can't go wrong with Martin's romantic comedy **Roxanne**, an excellent modern play on Edmond Rostand's 1897 play Cyrano de Bergerac (which is not to be confused with the early 1980s BBC crime drama series, Bergerac, with John Nettles as Detective Sergeant Jim Bergerac who solves crimes around Jersey), and the spectacularly stupid Carl Reiner classic, **The Jerk**, which has the sort of very silly laugh-inducing joke cavalcades in it that you almost feel guilty for chuckling at ("He hates these cans! Stay away from these cans!") as an idiot wanders out into the world to find his real family but accidentally finds riches and love 'by mistake'.

I admit that the term 'underrated' is very malleable when it comes to films and that's because our opinions around their quality are entirely subjective, aren't they? What I may consider "underrated" because it didn't do very well at the box office and not enough people liked it or remember it now, may have been perfectly received in your opinion because you didn't like it. For me though, these are the comedies that really make me laugh, take me away from troubled thoughts for a bit and can make me feel good but aren't as 'big' nowadays or simply weren't as big as they should have been when they were released.

The Hot Rock (initially released in the UK in 1972 as How To Steal A Diamond In Four Uneasy Lessons) is an effortlessly brilliant construction of multi-faceted comedy and crime caper, married together with an exceptional cast in which there's not a bum-note among any of them. The plot of the movie is pretty much covered in the UK re-title. It's a quiet masterpiece, frankly. Robert Redford, George Segal, Paul Sand and Ron Leibman are all truly brilliant. So much so that it says a lot about the fact that when Zero Mostel turns up (a man renowned for walking into films and stealing the whole shebang out from underneath everyone on the cast list, no matter how big) he actually has a fight on his hands to pull off stealing the picture this time around. This movie is a delight though - a director who knows how to construct tension even in the face of borderline slapstick comedy (That safety glass sequence? The safety deposit box finale?), Quincy Jones' soundtrack, a foursome who play brilliantly off one another and heist sequence upon heist sequence where you're caught hoping more and more goes wrong because you're enjoying hanging out with these characters so much... The only criticism to be levelled at this film is that it is too slight at just 100 minutes.

Remember earlier when I talked about childhood Saturdays spent taking the metro up to the local multiplex? **The Hard Way** is one of my fondest carryovers from that period. An action comedy about a grizzled New York City cop having to babysit a pampered actor who's studying him for an upcoming role all while trying to hunt down a crazed serial killer, I loved it as a kid and have only grown to love it more and more over the years. It's directed by John Badham, an underappreciated filmmaker whose films (Blue Thunder, War Games, American Flyers, Stakeout, Bird on a Wire) I grew up adoring and that guy can marshal one hell of an old school action sequence, which this is chockful of: Punch-ups, car chases, shoot-outs and that glorious Times Square climax... all married with some great laughs and an ace cast (Delroy Lindo, Luis Guzmán, Christina Ricci, Penny Marshall and Kathy Najimy to name but a few) doing brilliant work -

James Woods (replacing Gene Hackman) uses his intensity to an advantage, Michael J. Fox (replacing Kevin Kline) plays his role to pinpoint skewering perfection, Stephen Lang is terrifically bonkers and all but walks away with the film and, by God, Annabella Sciorra once again proves what an effortlessly astonishing talent she is. It's easy to make a good buddy movie. It's not so easy to make a great one yet this makes it look like it is.

Game Night is easily one of the greatest modern comedies of the last couple of decades. It is the story of a group of couples who get together weekly for 'game night' and suddenly find this week's meet-up hijacked by real life crime and intrigue they initially mistake for an elaborate 'game', and it has background / throwaway gags here that are stronger than most mainstream comedies best offerings (the whole 'Denzel Washington' thing, for example?) with a whole alternative entire 'mini movie' on a corkboard over the end credits with some top tier giggles that other comedy movies would be jealous of. It's a tight and impressively constructed comedy full of brilliantly staged and well-earned comedy set pieces stacked precariously on top of one another; each time one lands you think it's going to be the one that 'misses' and topples the movie and it never does. My 'happy place' nowadays remains watching this with my wife and watching her sob with laughter over the alleyway / gunshot scene.

The Wrong Guy is one of my favourite comedies of the 1990s and it is both bizarre and frustrating as to how underseen and underappreciated it is, mainly because of how poorly available it continues to be. It's so smart with its brilliant hook (what if an idiot thinks he's been accused of a murder he hasn't committed and goes on the run, but no one thinks he did it nor in reality is looking for him) yet so bloody silly and immensely assured in what it's doing. It's not spoofing those Hitchcockian type of movies. It's just gently nudging them in the ribs a little. Dave Foley is hilarious. There's some fantastic, hard laugh-out-loud moments and some truly terrific subtle, dry gags and it's all held together like super-glue by Foley's fully committed and on-point performance. There's jokes and visual gags here that are so pitch perfect in how they're executed and so unique that describing them would be fatal.

Admittedly very little of the once irritatingly prolific Judd Apatow's 'funny factory' stuff holds up these days but **The Forty-Year Old Virgin** – and the equally brilliant Knocked Up – certainly does. Tremendously so. In this movie's case (the title of which is the plot) it is because of the whole amount of heart that it has coursing through its veins alongside the profane and broad comedy stuff. Also, it has the platinum level secret weapon that is Steve Carell. With anyone else on screen and shepherding the script, this wouldn't be anywhere close to what it is. The gross-outs, coarseness etc aren't the foundation / drive of the film. They were almost the 'con' to lure you in (at a time when that sort of adult comedy sold big) so that you'll give this incredibly sweet film with a lovely message a chance.

It was a coin toss between **Kingpin** and Dumb & Dumber as to which of The Farrelly Brothers movies I included here. I love both of those movies dearly and both remain 'go to' medicines for some of that "natural antidepressant", and I feel I had to get The Farrelly Brothers represented in this chapter in some way because of how huge (and helpful) to me in my teenage years their work was when I needed respite from feeling so sad and lonely. Whilst I love Dumb & Dumber probably a little bit more on a personal level, I must acknowledge that this movie totally *kills* as a comedy. It's just so pleased with itself as to how wrong it is and how messed up it is prepared to get within the core structure of a sporting underdog movie – set within the competitive world of tenpin bowling. Yes, tenpin bowling. The jokes remain first class, the concept continues to be so bizarrely specific, and the performances are a joy across the board - Bill Murray absolutely nails it (which is not something you could say easily about him in broad studio comedies in the 1990s!), Woody Harrelson is fantastic, and Randy Quaid is positively sublime.

I've always found that in my lowest of moods the comedy films that have proven most effective in breaking through and getting me to laugh despite myself have been the more absurdist (i.e. stupidest and daftest) of films. And once they 'get you' good and start the chemicals flowing you can't help but come to appreciate the smarts and cleverness behind creating comedies this gloriously silly and cartoonish.

I remain steadfastly head-over-heels in love with Stephen Chow's **Kung Fu Hustle**. By gosh, it is an absolute piece of cinematic heaven; never to be equalled or even so much as replicated because it simply can't be (nothing Stephen Chow himself did before or has done since has come close). It's untouchable. It is so intrinsically its own thing, made by someone with such a specific clear and decisive vision as to what he wanted to achieve. I can still remember the first time I saw it I felt like I had no frame of reference for what it was I was experiencing - a live action Tex Avery cartoon by way of a wuxia action epic, whilst playing tribute to the Shaw Brothers kung fu films of the 1970s, acted out on one of the most impressive physical sets this side of Alfred Hitchcock's Rear Window. AND what's more it still makes me laugh uproariously to this day. It's impressive on a technical plane. It's immensely enjoyable on multiple levels as a martial arts movie too. And it's quite simply fantastic as a comedy.

I fail to understand why **InnerSpace** is not regarded as a masterpiece of the 1980s. When I think back to my childhood and my parents dumping me 'out the way' in front of some video tape, this is the film that jumps to the forefront of my memories, sitting cross-legged on the floor in the back room, watching this and eating Skips crisps. The story of a US test pilot shrunk down to cell size and accidentally injected into the body of a panicked hypochondriac, for its time and for what it's trying to achieve it is essentially a *perfect* movie! It hits every note as a comedy, as wild off-kilter sci-fi and as an action film - the first act is stupendously good in its execution; managing to introduce the two characters tightly, the pseudo-science the entire film needs to hang off AND roll into the second act with an exhilarating chase sequence. From there it's just relentless, unashamed fun with terrific action (the vehicle-to-vehicle escape sequence remains tremendously executed), wild set-pieces (the in-car fight between Martin Short and Meg Ryan and their recently half-miniaturised enemies is terrific) and very funny gags (basically everything Short does here is sublime). It's surprisingly touching too - there's life lessons to learn about true heroism being in all of us all along!

In a lot of ways, it is a miracle that **Step Brothers** works as marvellously as it does. Part of the Adam McKay / Will Ferrell 'quartet' made up of Anchorman: The Legend of Ron Burgandy, Talladega Nights: The Ballad of Ricky Bobby, this and The Other Guys (the last of which is *definitely* one of my absolute favourite comedies in the history of cinema and the only reason it isn't given proper inclusion here is because if I start waxing lyrical about its brilliance I won't stop), this film is such an almost *'Eh? What?'* of a concept – two middle-aged, emotionally stunted losers who still live alone with their respective parent are suddenly forced against their will to live together when said parent marries the other – and yet it works on every level for me (from the genius improv strokes through to the puerile brilliance of John C. Reilly's extended job interview fart). I get why some would find it irritating but, beat-for-beat, this is just splendid absurdism and character comedy taken to the extreme. (I remember feeling really low and sunken by another bad break-up and another round of abuse from my family, getting dragged to see this on opening night in 2008 by a friend who thought it might 'cheer me up', and the infectiousness taking hold from a sold-out audience screaming with laughter, clapping at punchlines and creating an atmosphere in and of the movie itself.) Far too late into my marriage I learnt my wife had never seen this film and I was insistent everything was dropped for this to be rectified. She was absolutely resistant to this demand - because *clearly* she has NO respect for the fuckin Catalina Wine Mixer - and was so unnecessarily agitated and po-faced towards this for its first stretch ...then she suddenly started to smile... then Will Ferrell's *"We'll have SO much more space for activities!!"* line broke through... and then the infamous bunk bed scene absolutely crippled her... because this is that sort of brilliant! You can fight against it – but it gets you!

Barb & Star Go To Vista Del Mar is one of the best comedies of the last decade (at the time of writing this). Smack bang in the middle of the Covid-19 pandemic this arrived as a remedy on par with the actual vaccines themselves. It is a joyous, unabashed, full lean into pure unadulterated, completely committed incongruity set against the normalcy of two middle-aged ladies taking a holiday together. It sets its stall out within mere minutes, letting you know you need to climb on board for the ride or take the exit ramp straight away. It's not going to be for everyone, nor does it seem to want to be - and those coming to it because it's from the ladies who wrote Bridesmaids (another excellent comedy) are going to be very disappointed / surprised / appalled / etc. Vanessa Bayer nearly walks away with the whole movie off just a couple of tiny scenes. She is genuinely hilarious and leaves you screaming for a 'Talking Club' spin-off movie or streaming show. It stacks itself so sky high with care-free comedic effort that when something clunks it's only a matter of seconds before something brilliant comes along.

Eric Sykes' **The Plank** is one of THE **all-time great** British comedies. My love for it only grows stronger the older I get, and I came to it as a young boy through my paternal grandfather with nothing but adoration from the get-go. This thing packs more outright gut-rippling laughs in its admirably compact 50 minute running time than comedies twice its length.

Sykes has crafted a film that <u>appears</u> to totally embrace outright silliness but there's an astonishing technical brilliance and choreographed physicality bordering on the genius lying behind said "silliness".

The comic potential - the *stratospheric* comic potential, no less - drawn from a plank of wood being handled by two workmen (and with little to no dialogue throughout) remains astounding.

Films As 'Bandages' Part II:

Films That Require You To Think And Help Distract

By now I feel my stall is well and truly set out in terms of arguing about films profound power to move you, transport you and even heal you. They can prove to be "natural antidepressants", as we discussed in the last chapter. They can inspire you and make you feel more hopeful in your outlook, as we'll look at in the next one. And they can make you think and challenge you to look at history from an alternative perspective or some of life's harshest of challenges with a different gaze. This last one is what we're going to look at a bit here.

Some people call them 'cerebral' movies.

They're the type of film that require you to invest and concentrate as opposed to switch on and passively watch. When watched in the right frame of mind as a mental health tool they can be *incredibly* effective. There's a reason after all when you start the talking therapies process you get asked questions on the Patient Health Questionnaire (known as PHQ-9 screening) and Generalised Anxiety Disorder form (referred to as a GAD-7 in medical settings) about how well you feel you can *concentrate* when watching a film or a television show.

The level to which you connect or can invest in a 'cerebral' movie is a useful indicator or barometer as to where your head is at and how in control of your thoughts you are – i.e. whether you can 'switch off' and concentrate on something else that requires it of you, leaving your present day thinking behind.

Aristotle believed an audience experienced a catharsis when watching the Greek tragedies; seeing characters facing dramas and challenges and empathising with them or seeing people in a story suffer hardships that made them sympathetic or even thankful that it wasn't happening to them. The recent boom in the true crime drama and documentary subgenres is said to stem from the emotional positions and vested interests it requests us to take in sympathising with victims and / or seeing justice achieved for them.

Films that require us to be challenged in our original stances or taken out of our present line of thought can be very powerful mental health tools. They can take us to a different emotional state from where we were before we watched them. They can even emotionally exhaust us to a level that they tackle our disrupted or disabled sleep patterns.

Historical dramas, crime thrillers and complex mysteries are frequently found to draw heavy feelings of intrigue, shock, fear, sadness, disgust, and other states that deeply affect us enough to pull us out of one feeling and into another if we're able to connect with the material, if only for the length of their running time.

And hey, we'll take *that*, don't you think? Who's looking for permanence at this point? A break from your 'racing mind' or negative ruminations will do for now.

I've mentioned my love for Sidney Lumet's The Verdict already, earlier in the book so taking that aside here's some films that I heartily recommend for helping you push yourself to invest in narratives and subjects that can assist in suspending overthinking and rumination. They're all complex, interesting films that I have found help to put some distance between me and my low mood or successfully measure where my mind is at in terms of my concentration levels:

David Fincher's **Zodiac** is an absolute favourite of mine and one of the great films to give yourself over to and be consumed by. It just gets better and *better* with each viewing too.

It is honestly an astounding and masterful piece of cinema with not a single weak moment or faltered minute in its whole running time! I get devoured by it every single time I watch it.

It's not a film you are casually entertained by whilst flicking through your phone, it's a modern cinematic classic and a work of *art* where everything is in the *details*. It's horrifying. It's thrilling. It has levity too. And it's one of the best films ever made about investigation - the passionate, tireless, often fruitless, sometimes obsessive, intricate art of investigation. It says everything that David Fincher made Se7en and Fight Club, both modern masterpieces of that there's no doubt, yet <u>this</u> is his best film.

Actor-turned-filmmaker Peter Berg may be seen as a bit of a joke to some people these days having disappeared down an 'American Heroism Seen Through The Perspective of Mark Wahlberg' rabbit hole, but that should not be allowed to distract entirely from the fact that he was responsible for **The Kingdom** - a brutal, slick as hell, effective mainstream thriller that still stands up as a bit of a near-masterpiece of its genre. Using the 1996 bombing of the Khobar housing complex, the 2004 Khobar massacre and the two 2003 bombings of four compounds in Riyadh as dramatic "*inspiration*" this is two-thirds truly brilliant investigatory procedural to one-third unreleased pressure valve of bombastic action and nerve-wracking tension. Its messaging occasionally stumbles into the sort of heavy-handedness you'd expect from Berg (the final denouement/epilogue is a clunker) and could be seen by some as wishful revisionism of the American response to Islamic fundamentalist in much the same way Rambo sequels were a fantastical bloodlust in the Vietnam War's aftermath. Take the film for its core intrinsic entertainment though and it is an absolute cracker; a perfectly paced, masterfully constructed, and remarkably satisfying action thriller.

I really do adore **Zero Dark Thirty**. It's a superb investigatory procedural about the real life intelligence-led hunt for Osama Bin Laden with that superb tension-drenched, dread-soaked covert operation attached on the back end. Sublimely perfecting the cinematic procedural last seen so well executed by David Fincher with Zodiac, Kathryn Bigelow has turned the said manhunt into an engrossing, exhilarating, fascinating, intelligent, thought-provoking piece of cinema. This came out of the gate as a ready-made modern masterpiece but US political figures clouded a lot of its excellence with debate and accusations around the issues on torture and its use / the part it played. The political noise doesn't dilute its power. There is a level of control on show here that marks Bigelow as one of the great directors of our time – She never lets the film get away from her and ascend to heady heights of overt-patriotism and overblown action set-pieces to pad out the sense of military might.

A recommendation of Sergio Leone's **Once Upon A Time In America** comes with a trigger warning for anyone who has been a victim of sexual assault. Now that the restored [2012 Cannes Film Festival] 251 minutes cut of it exists (overseen by Martin Scorsese's Film Foundation) and it is - due to unforeseen rights issues with regards to certain deleted scenes - the closest we will ever get to Leone's originally envisaged 269-minute version, it is the *only* version that should be viewed here on out. I'm also one of *those* who buys into the theory (endorsed by Leone himself, no less) that the entire film – an epic tale of crime and friendship - is an opium-induced dream with DeNiro's Noodles remembering his past and envisioning the future from the opium den in 1933 whilst hiding from the syndicate hitmen. I take a lot of heat from my geekier friends on this because to some it's the filmic equivalent of being a 9/11 truther / anti-vaxxer / conspiracy theorist. This is simply **one of the greatest epic crime dramas ever made**. There are charges of misogyny and offensiveness levelled against the film and that's no surprise for a film with not one but two rape sequences (the latter of which involving McGovern is genuinely sickening). But it is imperative that the treatment of women and the behavioural attitudes towards them is kept within the context of these specific characters in this specific story from this specific time; the film is an inarguably terrific, epic poem of brotherhood, ambition, betrayal, violence, lust, love, greed and... yes, opium-driven projections to a possible future in a mind's eye and a past etched into your core.

Seven Days in May has never felt more prescient than it does now. It's as important and thought-provoking today as the era in which it was made in whilst pointing a finger to the 'future'. Two of the greatest ever screen actors, directed by one of the best directors there ever was and with a script by Rod Serling of The Twilight Zone? This is as good as it gets, man. Upon its release, it was said that this – the story of an American military man uncovering a plot within his own armed forces to overthrow the President of the United States' government and seize control of the country – was "*fantastical*" in suggesting something like it could have ever occurred. Then in time we learn that director John Frankenheimer was getting inside advice on just how plausible it was by none other than JFK himself and his team and, best of all, this very thing nearly happened 18 months into President Trump's term. The idea that a political 'side' needs to "*steal*" or take dominance by '*any means necessary*'? The concept of the American constitution only serving a purpose when it fits? It is thought-provoking to watch this up alongside what is going on in America under a Trumpian landscape. Hell, double bill this with A Face In The Crowd and you've got a pretty exacting measure of how a vast amount of people view the state of affairs in the US today.

Prince of the City is a film I can barely watch anymore because I've worked in uniformed services and I've seen corruption at play and the corrupt rise whilst the honest fall. It all resonates a bit too hard for me but I'm going to recommend it all the same because it is an excellent film; a sumptuous, slow burning, positively majestic drama exquisitely crafted by one of the great American masters, Sidney Lumet. Based on NYPD Narcotics Detective Robert Leuci's real life, the film forms an official trilogy of sorts alongside The French Connection and Serpico - the former's real life disastrous bust is frequently named checked here and the events of the latter ostensibly set in motion this very film. A fascinating dramatic NYPD cinematic tapestry exists watching the three films together, with this as the concluding chapter. It is a *beast* of a film: a nigh-on three hour movie that survives on the complexity of twisted moral codes and human interaction. To say it's shaded in ways demanding of your attention is an understatement. It is kind of beauteous that the characters here that present as having the strongest or cleanest sense of integrity are the mobsters the dishonest cop protagonist moves in circles with. Here the protagonist is no hero, more a self-serving narcissist with a very confused moral centre. That the real life person (Leuci) would end up with such an aspirational, lengthy NYPD career after the way his fictional representative (Ciello) behaves here is staggering. The exchange presented in the film's quietly devastating ending ("What did you say your name was?" "Ciello." "Are you *the* Detective Ciello?" "I'm Detective Ciello." "I don't think I have *anything* to learn from *you*.") reveals a policing institute that took the corrupt cop who sold everyone out to offset his own perjury and re-presents him as a man of professional integrity then gifts him a teaching job within their academy!

In many ways **The Day of the Jackal** is one of the quintessential films I'm referring to in this chapter when it comes to complex and detailed movies that require you to invest in them over your own thoughts and distractions. I love it for all the reasons my wife struggled with it (sample quotes from her watching it: "Does it speed up?" "Does it get going any faster than this?" "Just be straight up with me coz I will nap on you if it doesn't!"): It's this purposefully slow and measured, *methodical* and painfully diligent procedural that plays like an ode to the power of investigation and chasing facts. It holds up tremendously and its sense of tension and escalation in everything from small two-person conversations to the final ten minutes itself is just spot on in its execution. There was a truly abysmal remake back in the 90s with Bruce Willis and Richard Gere (doing an "*Oirish*" accent!) that is well worth swerving. And a Sky TV adaptation in 2024 starring two of my most hated actors that I will never watch.

First Man is a straight-out-the-gate modern American masterpiece whose box office reception on release showed that - like with Warrior, The Thing and The Shawshank Redemption – not a lot of people know jackshit about great cinema from the get-go. This is an engulfing, fascinating and at times incredibly moving epic that procedurally does for deep dives on space exploration what Zodiac does for investigation, Zero Dark Thirty does for terrorism and Prince of the City does for corruption. It truly is an astounding piece of work that deserves to be held in the highest possible esteem. I still break into a smile thinking about the sheer cinematic exquisiteness of it all, how it uses sound to shred away at your senses and how, with the simplest of close-ups of a child's bracelet, it took a hammer to my emotional resolve and has me welling up even now thinking about it. It really is an absolute work of art that I champ at the bit to revisit the minute the credits roll.

The Prestige is Christopher Nolan's period drama about warring magicians vying to be seen as the greatest illusionist in the eyes of the public in 19th Century London – jealousy, ambition and science could well destroy them both in the process though. And that's all you need to know about the film. If you've never seen it before that's absolutely all you should know about it going in. It is a film that's narratively constructed like a magic trick, with a twist / reveal stacked on top of one another so that, quite literally, nothing is at all what it appears to be to you. It's a terrific film for forcing yourself to engage and get out of your head because it lures you into believing that you're going to be able to 'catch it out' and rumble the film's twist(s) before they land. I assure you, you cannot.

The Spanish Prisoner sits alongside Spartan (which is such a *great* movie too!) as David Mamet's masterpiece. It's a mesmerising, compelling experience where trying to appear clever and second guess it is an absolute impossibility. You know those movies where Trailer-Voice-Man tells us that "nothing is what it seems" and "nobody can be trusted" but then you go to see the movie and within minutes you're shouting out who the bad guy is and why? Well, *this* is the movie that those bad versions go to bed at night and dream of being. If nothing else, this film teaches us that we should never, never, never disregard those Japanese tourists we always see floating around our favourite landmarks!

Time travel movies by their inherent nature tend to be very silly or fall in on themselves. **Time Crimes** is one of the rare exceptions. It sits comfortably alongside Tony Scott's Déjà vu as one of the more interesting, if underseen, films on the subject. Taking almost everyday banality as a jumping off point the film follows a man who accidentally gets caught up in a causal loop and must set about stopping his other selves from continuing to exist. Devoid of both impactive budget and any special effects, writer/director Nacho Vigalondo creates a dizzying and disorientating, darkly comic affair that rewards you like a slot machine paying out in full for your devoted attention.

Speaking of **Déjà vu**, I am an enormous fan of the late great Tony Scott and it was a really distressing day when he took his own life because the man's output in the 1990s when I was just forming into a big movie geek in my mid-to-late teens had a massive effect on me. He was much mocked in that 2000-2010 period for his rebirth with the eclectic editing, film-stock bouncing style of filmmaking but to dismiss that period as in some way 'lesser' (and Domino is a very bad film!) would be to throw away Man on Fire, which many see as his masterpiece. It would also mean discarding this; a phenomenally well-made piece of entertainment and a ridiculously under-rated film as science-fiction goes. Normally with time-travel movies there's this whole *headache* of the filmmaker trying to do a load of heavy lifting to get you to buy into the whole '*concept*' they're trying to sell you on so that you'll sit with their version of time travel, and you'll accept the "ride" wholesale. The best time travel movies (Back to the

Future, Timecrimes, etc.) don't care about that angle - their attitude is one of stone-cold confidence in the pseudo-scientific waffle and they just assume such confidence will be infectious. This treats the time travel angle like it is just a side tool in this investigatory procedural / latent love story they're trying to tell, and Scott never looks back once to see whether you're buying what he's selling. He just takes you on a ride and a half.

Fritz Lang's 1931 German thriller **'M'** tells the story of a serial killer targeting children and the combining of police and organised crime infrastructures to hunt him down. It was one of the first 'procedural' films as we know them now within the thriller / drama genre and it remains a magnificent, enthralling and absorbing psychological study with a truly staggering performance from Peter Lorre. You're drawn in on both the 'hunt' for his character and the psychology that fuels him. Lang – a positively sublime filmmaker, as great as there ever was – fills his film with reprobates and scumbags across all platforms and sides of the law as a subtle but fitting slight against the country for destroying itself with the permittance of Nazism.

If, like me, you rather foolish went through a period where you ever thought Ralph Fiennes was a pretentious, overrated arse and Rachel Weisz an obnoxious, overbearing talent stretching mediocrity to its very limits than **The Constant Gardener** is definitely the flick for you! They deliver performances here that are opinion-changing in their exquisiteness, within a film that is still timely and thought-provoking. In the ever-excellent Bill Nighy, you also have one of the screen's best-ever representations of what *real-life* evil looks like! John Le Carré was rarely not excellent and therefore his novels made for terrific source material. This is one of the best adaptations of his work, telling the story of a British diplomat trying to get to the bottom of a corporate corruption scandal that may have led to his wife's murder.

Prisoners seems to have this sort of weird backlash of sorts against it nowadays and I can't seem to understand why. I like it a great deal. The problem with the film is that people are trying to build it up and put it alongside something majestic, mature, and exceptional like Fincher's Zodiac or Bigelow's Zero Dark Thirty when it just isn't *that* type of movie at all. It's a *potboiler*; an ode to the big ensemble studio thrillers of the 1990s - all grandiose themes, big stars doing hammy *swing-for-the-hedges* work, dry proceduralism and storytelling that just asks you to go with it and not question stuff too deeply. Because it's a bit silly and neat for more discerning crime thriller fans. It's extremely well-directed and thoroughly involving, a modern textbook example of how to make these sorts of films in fact. You don't put a movie like this up alongside those aforementioned movies. You lean it up alongside something like The Negotiator. And that's not dissing The Negotiator either. Because The Negotiator is bloody *tremendous.*

There are still people out there that consider **Klute** as some straight sexual thriller; a precursor to the Basic Instinct type of movie or something. It really is less a conventional thriller and more a deep, deep fascinating character study following a small-town detective (Donald Sutherland) who's searching for a missing man and his only lead is a hardened New York prostitute. But the most interesting character is not the detective but the character of the convention-bucking prostitute who refuses to capitulate to a single cinematic stereotype - and she's played by Jane Fonda with an intensity, ferociousness and strange vulnerability that rightfully shattered the expectations and opinions of nearly every critic on release. Part of Alan J. Pakula's '*paranoia*' trilogy, this would probably get written off by modern audiences now the minute they realise they're not seeing any of the murders or getting a lot of gratuitousness from the sex scenes. They would probably not accept that it is a 'thriller' on its own terms, not yours... and they'll probably not be around long enough to see Fonda, in all her teary and snot-strewn glory sit silently reacting to an audio recording of her friend in distress - subsequently delivering one of the greatest performances of the seventies in the process! And that's crazy and frustrating to me.

Of the 'Sherlock Holmes versus Jack the Ripper' films available (see also: A Study In Terror) **Murder By Decree** is the superior effort. It's the late Bob Clark's best work and the masterpiece within his filmography, a directing CV that is too easily written off as belonging to the "man behind Porky's". Christopher Plummer and James Mason offer up one of my all-time favourite incarnations of Sherlock Holmes and Dr Watson, respectively. I love their little comedic moments together (like their discussion as to the best method of picking peas up off the plate), as they investigate the murders of Jack the Ripper and uncover a conspiracy that reaches the highest society members in the country involving the sinister movements of the Freemasons and members of the Royal Family. I dig the hell out of this flick and I always get goose bumps in the film's final twenty minutes when Plummer's Holmes goes to a closed meeting with the Prime Minister (played rather woodenly by stage great John Gielgud), the Home Secretary and the Head of the Police and launches into his brilliantly-written, sublimely performed monologue of exposition that ties together everything we have previously viewed. ("I accuse...")

Night Moves is one of the best private investigator movies ever made. It's a labyrinthine crime thriller centred by one of Gene Hackman's best performances (and that's saying something seeing as the man was very *rarely* less than excellent in everything!).

The plot is a red herring drenched run around in the best possible way; it makes complete sense, it's just unashamed about being complex - refusing to allow us as viewer to be a step out of pace with Hackman - who every step of the way finds *something* forcing him to revise everything he thought he knew... right up to the end itself when we leave him behind, still putting the pieces together.

The last shot of the film is aerial coverage of Hackman's Moseby in an aimlessly circling boat and that's a pretty terrific metaphor for the guy's investigation we've just watched him try to survive. ("I didn't solve anything... This just fell in on top of me!") It's a motherfucker of a line that *nails* a tremendous film, one of the best of the 1970s, delivered by one of the greatest ever actors.

Master filmmaker or not, Steven Spielberg can fumble an ending and in the dying seconds of **Bridge of Spies** – the true story of an American lawyer tasked to defend an arrested Soviet spy in court then help the CIA facilitate an exchange for him with a captured US pilot – he drives his point home visually with a sledgehammer. Minor grumbles aside, this is the perfect storm of exquisite actors delivering a fascinating story through the lens of a master of cinema. The argument as to this being "*lesser Spielberg*" is a dud. The guy is playing around in his sandbox of skills and delivering an engrossing, surprisingly dry-humoured, atmospheric drama that ticks every box. There's nothing *lesser* about it.

Finally, **Killers of the Flower Moon** is simply astonishing to indulge in - there's such a deft, surprising *delicacy* to elements of this that's even more astounding considering the abhorrent subject matter.

That comes mainly from the performance Lily Gladstone provides this film with. In a sea of tremendous work - and by God it's both magnificent to see Robert DeNiro be great again and for Leonardo DiCaprio to *finally* do something in my eyes that lives up to his [overstated] reputation - she is working on some other stratospheric level.

Comments about this film's length by some don't resonate with me. I certainly didn't feel it, necessarily.

It's probably the length it needs to be to do justice to the masterful source material its adapted, deliver a legitimate love story (of which, don't be fooled by its toxicity, this *is*), a film of weighted historical and cultural context and a true life / true crime procedural.

It's surprisingly less gratuitous than you'd probably expect too. Especially considering we're in the hands of our greatest living filmmaker, someone who's never shied away from presenting us with absolute violence of an uncompromised nature.

This is a film that *consumes* you. It pulls you in and drags you down - you're in the presence of pure evil and weak character, and Scorsese expertly holds you there so escape feels as impossible as justice must have to the Osage. It's very easy to 'throw around' the term "*masterpiece*" when it comes to Martin Scorsese. Mainly because the guy keeps effortlessly making 'em. But by crikey this really is one.

Films As 'Bandages' Part III:

Films That Can Inspire and Make You Feel Good

If we've come this far than we have reached a point where we're willing to accept or at least consider the possibility that when it comes to our emotional well-being and mental health films can work as a "natural antidepressant" in terms of making us laugh and smile, as well as help distract ourselves or become mentally invested in something complex enough to draw us away from our state of negative rumination or worry – even temporarily. We're now going to look at the films that can make us feel emotionally warmed, hopeful, or drawn towards how we would *like* to feel.

When we watch films for these reasons, we do so with the latent aspiration of seeing someone we can empathise with and who goes on some sort of physical or poignant journey that ends in a way that we are left wondering even if ever so slightly that the same outcome could befall us. It's said that in a state of loneliness or recovery from a recent break-up romantic comedies are a type of film most people gravitate *towards*, not *away* from; wanting to see an idealised amorous connection that they can dream about for themselves going forward.

The two most common 'comfort blanket' types of films though remain films that show characters develop personal progression that puts them in a stronger / better state than they were when we first encountered them narratively and films that make us feel good and exhilarated, where protagonists go up against stacked odds and overcome them.

There are four types of movies of this ilk I want to spotlight for you in this regard. There's the character-driven stuff where the plot and / or the comedy is drawn from the human interactions. There's the romantic stuff that's healthy for your heart, trust me. Then there's the uplifting personal growth movies. And finally, there's the feel-good sports / underdog films that work like a shot of adrenalised serotonin to your brain.

Let's start with the character-driven stuff: I consider **Planes, Trains & Automobiles** to be one of the funniest films I've ever seen. I judge this on the grounds that I've seen it a ridiculous number of times, and I know what is coming through frequent viewing like I know the back of my own hand, yet I still laugh uproariously each and every time. It's the story of a man trying to get home to Chicago from New York for Thanksgiving and the overly helpful hinderance of a travelling salesman who keeps inadvertently hobbling his attempts. I would have included it in amongst the "natural antidepressant" selection of comedies were it not for the whole heap of heart it possesses. Heck, I feel so *seen* in John Candy's Del Griffith character that it nearly got an 'I Feel Seen' chapter all its own. It is a comedy seeping in confidence because, deep down, it knows that a truly great, timeless, effective comedy works on the theory that if it is perfectly cast and soundly constructed, then all else will flow naturally. And there is, it is said, nothing greater than a 'natural' comedy high. This film knows it has ticked all the right boxes and so it sits back and lets you come to it, instead of bouncing deliriously from weak gag to mediocre gag in need of your attention. This is touching, hilarious and genuinely magnificent piece of cinema that teaches you the importance of taking time to let people in, no matter how different they are to you, and learning to understand how another person feels.

For all the spoofing, aping, honouring and so forth, **The Shawshank Redemption** – a tale of friendship inside the walls of a sadistic prison, told over many decades - continues to age *tremendously,* doesn't it? It's an instant classic that holds its ground wonderfully. Litigation may have seemingly killed Frank Darabont's career (... or the leaked emails relating to The Walking Dead legal complications did!) but he remains an *incredibly* fine director who knows the value in casting talented people and getting out of their way. Less overtly emotionally manipulative than his equally brilliant follow-up movie The Green Mile, this is a film that as it develops you could pull a single thread and the entire preposterousness of the narrative could crumble, but no one ever does - because we *love* these characters so much and take this as less of a straight drama and more of a wondrous fairy tale fabling the might of the human spirit.

I truly believe Steven Soderbergh's remake of **Ocean's Eleven** is one of the modern greats - an exceptionally talented filmmaker bringing his love of European cinema and off-kilter narrative storytelling to a mainstream blockbuster, with fantastic results. He makes this Las Vegas heist movie feel so *effortless*. Nearly all of this cast, outside of Clooney / Pitt / Roberts / Reiner, were last minute *substitutes* for much more massive names (Elliott Gould jumped in for Michael Douglas at the last minute, Scott Caan and Casey Affleck replaced Owen and Luke Wilson, Matt Damon substituted Mark Wahlberg thankfully and Andy Garcia came aboard when Bruce Willis, Harrison Ford and Mel Gibson opted out of the Terry Benedict role because of the money) yet now they feel destined to have been put together all along. It's just so much *fun* and it's a movie that just slides by on a camaraderie and charisma that makes you feel like you're less a passive viewer and more an included member of the team.

I legitimately cannot speak highly enough of **Sing Street,** which is undoubtedly one of the loveliest, sweetest films you'll ever see. Whilst it gets lazily compared to The Commitments, I like it *more* – which is "sacrilege", apparently. This film plays like an autobiography of my teenage years if you replaced the musical aspirations with ones for writing and making films. It takes me back to one of the best summers of my life, hanging out for a couple of months with my friend Richard, making silly shit with camcorders and bit-by-bit other classmates slowly getting pulled in. Whenever I'm feeling low, I know that I can put this on and get a break from my present feelings by accessing very warm memories of mid-90s summers with my best friend and a camera making scene-for-scene remakes of the musical montages from Footloose just for the 'what-the-fuck-ever' of it (true story!) and realising it was one of the happiest parts of my adolescent life! The performances here are across the board brilliant, the soundtrack was as immense as any child of the 1980s would want it to be and it plays out ultimately as one of the best 'feel good' movies.

I quietly regard **Still Crazy** as one of my favourite comedies of the late 1990s and one of my favourite British comedies, full stop. The story of a 1970s rock band named Strange Fruit, who, after being split up for two decades, are persuaded to get back together despite hating each other, there's something incredibly *quaint* about this now - a film that delights in an almost unashamedly old-fashioned 'sitcom-esque' approach, which kind of makes sense when you note the screenplay is from Dick Clement and Ian La Frenais, the golden gods of the yesteryear TV sitcom format. It's great people (Timothy Spall in one of his last roles before losing the weight and going all serious, Withnail & I director Bruce Robinson in a rare acting part, Jimmy Nail just about hanging on in there, good ol' dependable Stephen Rea, Billy Connolly giving it the gold standard 'Billy Connolly' and Bill Nighy doing such wondrous things with the material here that Richard Curtis cast him in Love Actually and plagiarised most of the comedy beats from this) playing broad caricatures in a film correct in believing warmth will go far. And it *does*. Because as hacky and basic as it all is, such warmth is cultivated with these characters through this cast that the ending is a massive 'feel good' hug!

Based on Barry Crump's book 'Wild Pork and Watercress' Hunt **For The Wilderpeople** is about a reluctant father figure and a foster kid who become subject of a national manhunt after fleeing from social services into the New Zealand wilderness, and it is an absolute, total and utter, out-and-out delight. I adore it. The backlash against Taika Waititi is not *just* because he's overexposed but because he's overexposed due to believing his own hype. The man was at his best when his films carried the confidence of knowing the Kiwi sensibility and his off-kilter mining of it for humour was a goldmine that simply needed presented in this low-fi, matter of fact manner. He's at his worst currently (see JoJo Rabbit and Thor: Love & Thunder) because he's co-opted the Kiwi sensibility as *his* personality and he's cinematically two inches from your face now constantly screaming *"AREN'T I FUNNY? AREN'T I HILARIOUS? LOOK HOW WACKY I AM!"* Here though? Here he's just *perfect* in his handling of this material and his cast. It's hilarious, moving and gorgeously shot with a legitimately awards-worthy performance from Sam Neill that went completely ignored.

Onto the romantic stuff, and apparently men aren't *meant* to like **The Notebook**. Stuff that! It's wonderful. It's not just the two tiered performances with Ryan Gosling and Rachel McAdams breaking through the stratosphere with their charismatic, sensual, and warm turns whilst James Garner and Geena Rowlands shore up the back end with their deeply moving, lovely and human work together. It's not just the layered story either which realistically is nothing but a tired *"wrong side of the tracks" / "star crossed lovers"* tale with a highly emotional hook. It's the absolute, fully committed *sincerity* of it all. It strives to tell an old-fashioned story in an old-fashioned way, never once cow tailing to modern conventions or expectations or feeling like the tropes its playing with are beneath it or deserve to be side-eyed. It's just an incredibly, incredibly easy film to love - two hours of great actors doing great work, investing cheese with all the heart they're capable of and driving the whole thing through to a terribly affecting and lovely conclusion.

Defending Your Life – a fantasy involving a man who dies and is put on trial in the afterlife to examine all his fears and decide whether he is entitled to reincarnation back on Earth, only to fall in love with another soul during proceedings - is one of my go-to comfort movies. As a kid, I always wondered about what my notion of Heaven would look like and how you would have to 'earn' your place there. (Hey, I got in early on the dark depression thing, what can I say?) Albert Brooks kind of *nails* envisaging it for me. In the process he's made a very funny and oddly comforting movie, with a delightful performance from Meryl Streep in one of my favourite roles of hers. Everyone should experience this film at least once in their life. You become all the better for doing so.

Only Rob Reiner walked away from **When Harry Met Sally** with the strength to keep his legendary 'run' as a filmmaker going (seriously, go back and look at that eight year run from 1984 to 1992!). Nora Ephron never wrote anything as brilliant as this again. Meg Ryan was never more delightful than she was here. Whilst Bruno Kirby and Carrie Fisher ultimately sneak scenes out from underneath her, this is absolutely her film through and through. Billy Crystal would come close to equalling his appeal and comedy zest here with City Slickers a couple of years later, but in reality, he was never as good again as he was here. The perfection of this film *drained* them. And it *is* a perfect film. A masterclass in not letting ego nor the 'page' get in the way of what is best - because what's best about this film, the story of whether a platonic friendship between a man and a woman will become something more, comes from the core contributions of one and all. Don't believe it? The infamous deli zinger ("*I'll have what she's having!*") was a Billy Crystal suggestion that he pushed Rob Reiner to give to his mum, who was working as an extra in the background! The insert interviews of real life married couples were something the legendary Carl Reiner told his son he should scatter amongst the film as 'chapter headings'! Most of Crystal's more miserable lifestyle traits came from Carrie Fisher's real life behaviours! There's a reason this film remains so repeatedly and relentlessly pillaged from within the romcom genre even to this day – it's because it is a masterpiece!

I have a deep, deep, unbridled, and unashamed *love* for **Muriel's Wedding**, quite simply one of the best uplifting personal growth movies ever made. It is a movie that, like the best in Australian cinema, uses the colourful kitschy backwater aura to lure you in with the notion you're here to laugh at these broad Aussie caricatures... then it hits you with something of real *depth* and *emotion*. This is a film that is funny on face value but incredibly moving under the surface. It's about the intense and immense *power* that comes from marrying the realisation of your own worth with the value of a deep and true friendship. I say this with zero hyperbole whatsoever; Toni Collette gives, for me, one of the *greatest* performances of all time here... *Of. All. Time.* She changes her character's weight, gait, sexual confidence, attitude, and dress throughout in such a way that you could easily believe an entirely different actress is playing Muriel by the film's end than who portrayed her at the start. Right behind her is Jeanie Drynan who gives one of the most severely pained, internalised and profoundly moving performances I've ever seen - I've never seen anyone act before in such a way they could make my eyes well up just from how they slowly drop their head at a dinner table, conveying decades of unspoken hurt and repression in the process. And all of this makes it sound like an incredibly *harrowing* film, I accept that. That it isn't, that it manages to also be so frequently funny, delightful, and inspiring too speaks to the film's true brilliance.

Cameron Crowe means so much to me now because of how much he once meant to me way back when. He may well be decidedly off the boil and culturally 'out of favour' currently but I'll always hold a massive place in my heart for him and what he made me feel as I was growing up. It's so easy to forget now because of the generational shift and how he's become such an uninspired hack of sorts, but there was a time when that guy's cinematic voice was a lifeline for people like me. His debut Say Anything is one of the greatest movies (let alone teen movies) ever made and helped navigate me through my difficult high school years. Singles, his 'difficult second movie', was seen by me too young for it to resonate initially but by crikey did it land just right when I hit my mid-twenties and started trying to find my way through love and life. Almost Famous stands as both a modern classic and one of the greatest acts of 'cinema as autobiography' we've ever seen. And, of course, there's **Jerry Maguire**. We're quick to forget now but it was *massive* and is just such an unashamedly pure and earnest 'swing for the backboards' the likes of which would never ever get made by a major studio today (and we're talking about a $273 million success story off a $50 million budget). It's a movie about a sports agent in emotional and professional crisis, and yet somehow resonates in one way or another with each of us.

People have seemingly softened on **Stranger Than Fiction** over the years, but I've held fast in my adoration of it. Maybe the high concept (a man's mundane life is thrown off-kilter when it becomes narrated by a voice only he can hear – and when the voice declares he is facing imminent death he realises he must change his fate and challenge the 'story') has worn off for some people? There's just something about it that hits me and works on a deeply personal level. The acting is very nearly uniformly excellent - it hurts seeing Dustin Hoffman be so effortlessly brilliant here with so little, knowing we've as good as lost him professionally forever now. The weak link here is Maggie Gyllenhaal; an actress whose very voice and purposefully over-earnest choices just grate on me. She's completely wrong / insipid here. The film overall though is a profoundly moving, interesting and surprisingly funny film - and in the case of the latter, not *at all* in the way you'd expect for a Will Ferrell movie. (He gives a career best performance here).

I was once indifferent to **Nobody's Fool**, but it grows *with* you and it communicates things to you if you allow it to. It's a big, warm embrace of a film that teaches you the grandest richness lies in our human connections and how it is never too late to change the lot that life has given you. It's the sort of unshowy and unpretentious movie that rewards you for sticking with it past its wobbly opening - where characters speak initially like stage-play characters instead of human beings - by giving you a magnificent Paul Newman performance (was there ever anything else?) backed by a delightful turn by Jessica Tandy. It's just a lovely, nice, moving and quite inspiring little film. One that really does serve to remind you that Newman was a master at this lark. He really made it look so *natural*.

I was absolutely, unequivocally obsessed with John Badham's sporting underdog movie **American Flyers** as a child and I consider it to be one of the greatest sports movies ever made now. In the world of such films (certainly cycling films) it is an absolute *tour de force* of feel good exhilaration. The story of two brothers facing down family tragedy by teaming up to tackle the most gruelling sports event in professional cycling, Kevin Costner and David Grant are a wonderful pairing and make the soapy subplot something that's actually *really* moving and lovely, soundtracked by Greg Mathieson and Lee Ritenour's incredibly unsung synth-tastic, adrenaline-pumping musical score. There's even a bit where one of the *actual* stunt riders takes a corner too fast and *actually* goes off an *actual* fuckin cliff and, shitteth ye not one jot, they leave it in the *actual* film. Seriously. This is just a great time, man. When I was a kid, I visited the local video shop so often they gave me my own "*junior card*" because I spent every Saturday riding my bike over there to obsessively stare at all the cover art before choosing a film. (I basically used it to rent the *same* five films over and over again: this, Rocky IV, The Princess Bride, The Monster Squad and Big Trouble In Little China!) A big, broad, high cheese, fist-pumping slice of feel-good perfection. There's that entire 'Breakaway' sequence which is so well executed and exhilarating it is like you've been injected with a shot of *pure* adrenaline. Then there's the finale with the clock counting down and the slow motion and the searching for each other in the crowd and... no, *YOU'RE* welling up, you big soft arse!

What can possibly be said about **Rocky** that's not been said already by everyone? No matter the sequels and the spin-offs, this still stands as one of the best feel-good-movies America has ever made since Frank Capra stopped making them. One in which the behind-the-scenes rags-to-riches stories (regarding unbankable and unknown writer/star Sylvester Stallone holding firm on starring in the script he'd written) are as good as the film itself, turning this tiny $1 million 'indie' into a $100 million box office and cultural sensation. The movie is extraordinary because it wants to involve us on a simple, take-at-face-value level. It takes the notion of heroism and realising your potential, about taking your best shot and avoids being corny by really working on those levels. If you are truly honest with yourself Rocky only feels cliched to those bored of montages, big final fights, post-punch up declarations etc. all recycled to the point of exhaustion *since* this film. Unlike with the rip-offs and a few of the sequels, we truly care about this character as if he exists: When Rocky delivers his speech about wanting to "go the distance", we sincerely want this character to achieve the greatness he yearns for because we feel he has earned it.

Warrior is one of THE great modern American movies. It's a new generation's The Shawshank Redemption in the sense that we all slept on that goddamn movie initially too only for it to be swiftly recognised as a masterpiece. It is a film of such ferociousness and yet also surprising delicacy about two estranged brothers both at difficult points in their life for different reasons and forced to enter a big pay-out MMA (mixed martial arts) tournament to try and survive, only to end on a collision course towards one another. Forget all this "*new Rocky*" or "*Rocky for the MMA crowd*" bullshit. This is so not that. It's instead a quiet story of forgiveness and redemption. It's also subtle study of PTSD and addiction. It's a humane look at the sins of the father upon his sons. Every moment of it feels real and painful and inspiring and moving. The film builds to an atypical 'sporting underdog movie' conclusion then uses it as a canvas on which to paint resolution and rectification between two brothers. If you're at this tear-inducing climax (and by the time Mark Isham's score slides into The National's beautiful song as the camera finds Nick Nolte's face in the crowd, you'll be sobbing) still thinking you favour one brother over another here you've not been watching it right: It doesn't matter who "*wins*" the fight. If these two characters can find their way back to one another after decades estranged than they've both won, really.

We've become so cynical and so abrasive towards a feelgood movie experience that letting one 'in' seems a rare, standalone experience nowadays. Our cynicism is so entrenched that it appears to have killed that entire subgenre of live action true life sporting underdog movies they don't seem to regularly make any more. I'm *big* on those films Disney had cornered the market on; the likes of McFarland USA, Secretariat, Remember The Titans, The Rookie, Cool Runnings, the underrated gem that is Glory Road and, of course, the masterpiece of the form that is **Miracle**. (Only Invincible is a bit rubbish!) I used to never really understand why they gave up on them... other than the very real possibility they'd ran out of true life sporting underdogs to portray... and then it became apparent that it was our *cynical apathy* towards them that killed the subgenre. Here's a film that lifts and runs with the Disney template to thoroughly enjoyable and wonderful effect. Director Gavin O'Connor knows he has the goddamn story of stories when it comes to underdog tales with this recounting of how the legendary Herb Brooks led the 1980 USA Olympic hockey team to victory over the seemingly invincible Russian squad by rostering the team with unknown college athletes. And he goes deep on maxing out the authenticity so that even at the most incredulous of feelgood moments a quick fact check swiftly reveals "Holy shit! This Brooks fella and these lads really *did* do [this or that] and then pull this off!"
I *still* find it insane that Disney never even bothered with an awards season

push for this film AND for Kurt Russell, who should've got an Oscar nomination for his work here (hell, Kurt Russell should've won many Oscars full stop). The real life Brooks died in a car accident half a year before the movie was released. Allegedly on his way to see the first cut of this very film, no less. At the end the title card states: *"This film is dedicated to the memory of Herb Brooks. He never saw it. He lived it."*

The Cutting Edge is such a totally underrated gem of a film - so incredibly likeable, enjoyable and really rather sweet. It's funny, romantic, and involving with a great soundtrack and a performance by Moira Kelly that is one of the most unjustly unsung in the romcom genre. It's just got one of those sort of wonderful log-lines where the minute you describe it - a boorish, injured hockey player and a prima donna champion figure skater have to team up to compete in the Olympics together - you can see the smile break-out on the face of the person you're describing it to as they go "Okay, I admit that sounds stupid, sweet and rather fun!" And it is.

To me **Major League** is a perfect construction; one of the greatest sports movies ever made. David S. Ward has written and directed a film that is just joyous to experience - he's crafted a legitimately solid underdog comedy, got the bawdy tone for it just right and fleshed it out with genuinely loveable characters you really want to see come good (even the purposefully dickish ones) up against a grand panto-esque villain, deliciously played to the hilt by Margaret Whitton. Ward has laid steel strong foundations with his script and then cast sublimely on top of it. This thing is so good that it even elevates Charlie frickin Sheen, man. Ward doesn't cast big. He casts talent that can bring these characters to life. It's no wonder the likes of Rene Russo, Wesley Snipes and Dennis Haysbert broke big from this. And they're positioned alongside absolute pitch-hitters like Tom Berenger, Corbin Bernsen, James Gammon, Chelcie Ross and Charles Cyphers as well as a scene-stealing Bob Uecker. About an hour in there's *that* scene... ("Well then I guess there's only one thing left to do." "What's that?" "Win the whole fucking thing.") ... and the film just *takes off*

- set against James Newton Howard's score, it's an extended montage into one of the most dramatic, fantastically structured, feel good climaxes in sporting movie history. We've come to really care about the likes of Berenger's broken down, over-the-hill Jake Taylor (even if his pursuit of Russo's Lynn Weslin *is* highly questionable looked at by today's standards) and we need to see him get what he deserves. This still stands as one of the funniest, most perfectly etched comedies of the 1980s and of all time.

I read an article online a few months back, some think-piece op-ed thing about "problematic, lazy representation" in cinema and **Cool Runnings** was high up on the list of examples and my genuine first thought was "Cool Runnings? You're coming after Cool Runnings? Why would you want to cancel Cool Runnings? It's... It's... *Cool Runnings*?" It is funny and enthralling and sweet, and exactly the sort of warm live action sporting underdog stuff we deserve more of - big, broad, swing-for-the-fences inspiring cheese with grand speechifying and stirring Hans Zimmer scores – with a reckless fealty to actual 'truth'. The equally lovely and delightful Eddie The Eagle would utilise its template to great effect many years later. It becomes obvious what a huge miss John Candy remains whenever you go back and watch one of his films. He was an effortlessly funny and charismatic man. What he never got enough credit for to his dying day was what a wonderful dramatic actor he was too - whether it's in that delightful bit with Keri Green on the beach in Summer Rental or the entire back third of Planes, Trains & Automobiles. Or all of his scenes with Jean Louisa Kelly in Uncle Buck and Ally Sheedy in Only The Lonely. He's great here too. His final 'gold medal' speech with Leon is up there with all those aforementioned films.

I can't think of a more quintessentially 'atypical rainy Bank Holiday Monday' moment for any lad growing up in the 1980s then watching **Escape To Victory** with your Grandad and getting to THAT moment. You know the moment, *right*? It's the height of World War II and a group of Nazi officers have come up with a propaganda event in which an all-star Nazi team will play a team made up of Allied prisoners of war in a football game to be broadcast around the world. The prisoners agree, initially planning on using the game as a means of escape from the stadium mid-game. And here they are - it's half time, they're 4 - 0 down having faced the reality of dirty German tactics and a corrupt referee but none of that matters because the tunnel inside the changing room has successfully blown and the resistance is there to lead the POWs out. They're *FREE*. Then right there in that moment one of the players cries out: "Hang on a minute. We've got to go back. We can win this thing." Bill Conti's terrific score - all heavily lifted from the first and last movements of Dmitri Shostakovich's Leningrad Symphony - *swells up* and the POWs charge back out, realising that defeating the might of the Germans in front of the world matters more than their own freedom. And there's really nothing quite like it for taking you right back to your childhood and making the hair on the back of your neck stand up. There's a sense memory that can't quite be beaten in revisiting Luis Fernandez (Pelé), Carlos Rey (Osvaldo Ardiles) and Terry Brady (Bobby Moore)'s stunning goals. For too long this film was treated like some sort of dismissible kitschy joke because of the point it landed in (the immensely overrated) Michael Caine's much-mocked shitty career period and because of the whole (admittedly pretty rubbish) Sylvester Stallone '*doing Rocky as a goalie*' thing but it's no joke. It really isn't. It's a big hunk of old-fashioned 'man' movie, built up from the most reliable parts of beloved genres and subgenres; one part war movie, one part sporting underdog drama, one part escape thriller. It's not out to compete for your affection for The Great Escape. It's just out to entertain. It's so good to see it now start to get reappraised for the slice of joy that it really is - you don't need to write the whole film off because the Stallone thing is very dumb, and Caine looks ridiculous when he runs.

Finally, we've looked at some films that I recommend within the described categories but there's one movie I highly advocate that actually fits the criteria of being *all* of these types in one – a character-driven, romantic, sporting underdog movie all about uplifting personal growth that gives you a lovely shot of adrenalised serotonin to your brain. I mentioned it whilst discussing The Best of Times, but it is Ron Shelton's **Tin Cup**.

Many people seem to prefer Shelton and Kevin Costner *other* sports n' romance collaboration (Bull Durham) but to me I absolutely favour this - an all-time favourite of mine when it comes to needing something that ticks the box of feel-good comedy, sporting underdog drama and warm-hearted romance. It's frankly a *faultless* movie - for what it is and for what it is trying to be; a big ol' proverbial cuddle of a film that touches on masculinity, vulnerability, chasing greatness, self-reflection and "big swings" in both life and sport as a washed up golf pro working at a dead-end desert driving range sets about trying to qualify and win the US Open so he can prove his worth and earn the love of his rival's girlfriend. Rene Russo was a last minute draft pick and that seems insane now such is her incredible chemistry with Costner. The film is one of those joyous occasions when all sublimely crafted parts come together perfectly; Shelton has proven already that he can do this effortlessly, so his direction is relaxed and confident because he knows he's got a great cast and a terrific script of his own creation full of beauteous 'Sheltonisms' ("Sex and golf are the two things you don't have to be good at to enjoy!" / "When a defining moment comes along you define the moment or the moment defines you.") The secret weapon here is that you can take the film however you like and you're still going to find yourself incredibly rewarded, whether that's as a character piece about finding your worth, a late stage romance that feels very much real in the way the characters bounce off one another or as a sporting underdog yarn with THAT ending that circumnavigates the expected 'big win' climax with [something different] wrapped in William Ross' sumptuous, stirring score.

The Film Guide

Films You And I Can Bond Over

Die Hard

The Verdict

The Last Starfighter

Flash Gordon

Running Scared

Escape From New York

Welcome To The Dollhouse

Midnight Run

Ricochet

The Best of Times

Bird on a Wire

The Life Aquatic With Steve Zissou

The Prisoner of Second Avenue

Pee Wee's Big Adventure

The Rocketeer

The Package

Films That Can Make You Laugh

Airplane

This Is Spinal Tap

Stripes

Real Life

The Odd Couple

What's Up Doc?

City Slickers

Roxanne

The Jerk

My Cousin Vinny

Tootsie

The Hard Way

Game Night

The Hot Rock

The Wrong Guy

The 40 Year Old Virgin

Kingpin

Inner Space

Kung Fu Hustle

Dumb & Dumber

Step Brothers

The Other Guys

Barb & Star Go To Vista Del Mar

The Plank

Films That Require You To Think And Help Distract

Zodiac

The Kingdom

Zero Dark Thirty

Once Upon A Time In America

Seven Days in May

Prince of the City

The Day of the Jackal

First Man

The Prestige

The Spanish Prisoner

Time Crimes

Déjà vu

'M'

The Constant Gardener

Prisoners

Klute

Murder By Decree

Night Moves

Bridge of Spies

Killers of the Flower Moon

Films That Can Inspire and Make You Feel Good

The Shawshank Redemption

Planes Trains & Automobiles

Ocean's Eleven (2001)

Sing Street

Still Crazy

Hunt For The Wilder People

The Notebook

Defending Your Life

When Harry Met Sally

Jerry Maguire

Stranger Than Fiction

Nobody's Fool

Muriel's Wedding

Rocky

American Flyers

Warrior

Miracle

Major League

Escape To Victory

Cool Runnings

The Cutting Edge

Tin Cup

“Yippee Ki-Yay”

There may well *appear* to be some arch hypocrisy in me saying that the manner in which I finally tackled my mental health (in a way that I gained control over it for the first time in my *forties*) was through prioritising other people, more so when I’ve spent this book saying it’s about *you*, it’s *your* fight and giving you a detailed account of how I broke free from the emotional stranglehold of my family when I realised how toxic they were to my health. But this book has been about unvarnished truth so there’s no point lying to you as we cross the finish line together.

The truth is that whilst I had to learn to recalibrate my personal sense of self-worth and stop caring about what others thought or wanted of me, the only successful route to getting to a healthy place where I could gain control of my mental health and wellbeing was when I started thinking about what legacy I wanted to leave behind for my boys and how I felt deep shame and pain at the thought that if I left them by committing suicide they would think it was because I didn’t want to be in their life when in fact the *opposite* could not be more true.

I had spent my entire life up to this point chasing this ‘great’ moment.

I’ve wasted so much time and energy striving to achieve greatness by someone else’s standard then I had children and one day simply, quietly realised that *they’re* my great achievement.

And I’m a good dad to them.

I’d *like* to be a great one, but I need to get better at not projecting my anxieties and fears onto them, I can see that.

Nothing makes me wake up in a cold sweat at night, gasping for air, quite like having nightmares at the idea of either of my boys experiencing even a small percentage of the bullying I endured in my lifetime.

You start to think about what you want to leave behind for your kids, not just materially but as a legacy.

That thinking led me to carrying out a coup d'état on my mental well-being and eventually writing this book.

I wanted to get better with regards to my mental health *for them.*

And as a thank you to my wife for saving my life and protecting me so vehemently at the lowest and most mentally exposed period in my life.

Then right at the moment I started writing out some sort of rough draft plan as to how I was going to do it for them, I realised that I wanted it for *myself* just as much.

I wanted to know what a life could look and feel like for me when instead of always seeing the 'black cloud' looming up ahead, I am looking back at it, knowing it's there, keeping it in my sights, whilst quietly whispering "I see you. Stay where you are, motherfucker!"

All our journeys towards gaining a better understanding – and with it a better sense of control – of our mental health are obviously very different and very individual, but I hope in telling you my story there's things you can perhaps empathise with or see elements of that are at least slightly similar to something you're feeling or experiencing.

Or at a push can be stretched to fit.

My work stresses are not yours, but you could possibly apply what I'm saying to the type that you're having.

My family situation is different to what you've perhaps experienced, but the lessons I've drawn from surviving that childhood could be applicable to you in another capacity.

My aim has been to make whatever you're feeling seem a little less heavy and for you to look at your mental health differently; that you don't have to beat it, you can just learn to control it.

Think of it as 'brain mould', remember?

I want you to know that you can do this by not looking at the return of a low period in your emotional well-being as a 'failure' on your part to combat it.

Instead address its return by doing very small things day-to-day that can put distance between your feelings and your reality, between the influence the 'black cloud' has over you and the power *you* have over *it*.

And by changing your outlook or opinion on the strategies that are out there in the arena of mental health support.

Together, we've put forward some ways to go about exploring your attitude towards both therapy and antidepressants, and your relationship to them.

We've discussed learning to slow things down and to deal with 'this' and then 'that', to challenge our negative thoughts by requiring facts and evidence to be attributed to each of them, to set ourselves small goals that are intrinsically individual to us and to look at how we schedule and utilise our time to be able to have the space to work on them.

We've talked about having a little bit of a think around how you start your day, your connections with other people and your relationship with exercise in even its most *minor* of forms.

We've looked at the requirement to be self-reflective whilst being firm but fair to yourself and to proactively effect change then wear your experiences, good and bad, with a degree of pride.

Most importantly of all, we have shone a light on looking at what makes you happy and embracing that wholeheartedly. And we've really went *all in* on using movies as medicine, of course.

After all, the principles of what I've talked to you about from my own personal experience throughout this book are all right there in the major motion picture masterpiece Die Hard, aren't they? Let's drop back to that film one final time:

John McClane is trapped inside of the LA skyscraper that is Nakatomi Plaza on Christmas Eve, remember?

He's taking on terrorists (who are actually robbers!) and acting as an intermediary to the police outside whilst trying to save his wife, protect the hostages and keep himself alive.

He's looked at the situation and decided that he has to act because he doesn't know that he can depend on anyone else (**'Challenging the Catastrophe'**), he's taken out a pen and started to scribble on his arm to set himself targets and keep track of his goals – i.e. how many people he has left to kill (**'I Wasn't Aiming For You – Goals, Targets, Etc.'**).

He's reached out to Sgt Powell as a confidante and a means of support (**'The Cost of a Text'**) and they've been honest and vulnerable with each other in their communication (**'It's Good To Talk': Therapy and You'**).

McClane's then done some self-surgery on himself both figuratively and literally in the way that he's bandaged his gashed feet and come to accept that he has not been fair to his wife (**'Removing The Tumour: Self Surgery / Proactive Problem Solving'**) and he's managed his time effectively in order to combat the bad guys before they get away with the contents of the Nakatomi vault (**'The Compartmentalisation of Time Method'**).

Most importantly he's worked on only the adversity in front of him.

Dealing with the likes of Franco, Tony, Alexander, Kristoff, Heinrich, Fritz, Uli, and James (Eddie got punched out by Argyle, he doesn't count!) one at a time or in as small a set of groups as possible.

Until he was eventually in a strong enough position to brutally fight it out with Karl and then finally drop Hans Gruber off the building (**'The 3 T's Strategy'**).

By the end, McClane has survived the night, come to realise what's important to him is bigger than his resentment around his wife's career move and he's reunited with her and met Powell in person for the first time (**'Embracing The Small Stuff: Finding Joy'**).

At the risk of appearing *wildly* pretentious and analogically uncouth, my hope is that this book becomes like 'The Underground Railroad' for people struggling with their mental health.

In a similar way that said 'Railroad' was a whispered network of secret routes and safehouses that were used to get enslaved African Americans into free states and then on to Canada, I want this to be a guide that's recommended from friend to friend or counsellor to patient, even loaned out in dog-eared form from being read so many times (if you're happy that the restriction in royalties from lending out one copy instead of having others purchase their own is essentially *stealing the food from my children's' mouths*, of course!), as a source of support they'd possibly not heard of during difficult times:

"Psst, I can see you're struggling. Let me ask you this, have you heard of The Yippee Ki-Yay Principle?" or "Did you know Die Hard can be used as *therapy*?"

I wrote this book for my two boys.

It took a while for me to get over this deep fear I have that their abundance of love and respect for me will fade the older they get, and they will come to regard me the way so many others have treated me in my life or see me as this 'joke' that others do.

As much as I wanted to write a book that can help other people who have struggled with their mental health like I have, I also wanted to write a book that my boys can one day read and see that their ol' dad has done some "cool shit" and been through some "bad shit", but he never gave up even on his darkest day... because all roads were leading to *them*.

Maybe they'll grow up with a clear understanding of why I'm so very passionate about them liking what they like and embracing what they enjoy – even if some of their choices of entertainment at the time of writing completely bewilders me in all the ways I imagine Pee Wee's Big Adventure and Wayne's World befuddled my grandparents.

I love you both so much, boys.

You make me so incredibly proud that I get to be your dad. And if either of you are reading this it means you're now old enough to do so. Which likely means you both owe me money for *something*.

So, cough up. Let's not make it awkward.

I hope by talking about my experiences and sharing with you some things that have worked for me I have helped you in some way.

Even slightly.

If just one method discussed here or one film recommendation has 'lightened your load', made you feel a little better or helped you have your first good day in a while than that means the world to me, if I'm honest.

I guess you could say I've been the... no, wait... come back...

I guess you could say I've been the Sgt Al Powell to your Detective John McClane. No?

No?

Okay.

Well now you've made it awkward.

We're leaving things on an uncomfortable note now. Like one of those dates where you think it's gone well so you lean in to kiss the other person goodbye, and they quickly raise their hand up for you to shake instead.

Let's just leave it.

No, seriously it's fine. I'm sure this embarrassing bit won't survive the final draft anyway, right?

After all, who'd seriously end a book like this? I mean, c'mon...

"... They fuck you up,
your mum and dad.
They may not mean to,
but they do.

- Philip Larkin
'This Be The Verse'

Acknowledgements

It seems trite to say it but it is true none the less – without my wife there's no book, that's been true of the other three books I've written and it's even more so in this case:

Without her gifting me the children that inspired *this* book to be created, without her as a sounding board, fact-checker and occasional "Woah, that's too raw. I don't think you should put that out there!" klaxon-call you would not be holding this in your hands right now. There'd be nothing there. Just you, holding an imaginary book, looking weird. So, *you* have my wife to thank too.

I want to thank my two boys who will one day be old enough to read this and if ever they themselves have a day in their life where they're feeling a bit low or lacking in esteem / worth, they can look to this book and realise that they are so special and wonderful that they drove it into creation.

Its existence will hopefully be something that other people draw help and support from.

That's on *them*.

They should feel very proud.

A massive thank you also to Mark Flaherty who's patience, kindness and talent put this book across the line and into your hands with the magnificent cover-work adorning it. He's really *something* and I don't care where you are in the world, if you're requiring graphic design work of any kind you should check out his company Me & Alan.

With each of the previous books I've written I've always had a small 'cabal' of what I call "constructive readers".

These are people who read my second draft and give me feedback or corrections, sometimes shifting my work in different directions through their input (my second novel, Lehman's Run, had a drastically different and darker ending until one such constructive reader proffered platinum-tier opinions on it!).

This time round I wasn't just dependent on such people but I was reliant on those around me sharing their own mental health experiences and woes, putting me in touch with people in their own circle who were struggling or who had struggled, working to connect me to medical professionals or materials that would be useful too.

I can't thank those people enough in helping me put some 'weight' behind my text and for being wholly honest and giving to me about the difficulties in their lives.

I want to especially give a humungous thank you to Daniel, Katie, James and Amy who read this in various ugly states and cheered it across the finish line.

Finally, alongside both of my in-laws for their kindness / friendship / patience / tolerance, I want to thank **you** for taking the time to read this book and hopefully recommend it on to others who you think may find it useful.

The Yippee Ki-Yay Principle as I've outlined it here is a proverbial 'ladder' and we must always pass it back down to help lift others up and away from darkness.

That's the underpinning rule at the core of this book and, now you've read it, whether you like it or not you're part of the 'solution' going forward.

Take care of yourself. And each other.

Remember: *You are not your worst day!*

Leonard McClane

Copyright

The Best of Times is a 1986 motion picture created by Ron Shelton for the production companies Kings Road Entertainment, Inc. and Cinema Group Venture and it is directed by Roger Spottiswoode. It is owned by Kings Road Entertainment, Inc., Cinema Group Venture and Universal City Studios, Inc. Its Copyright Number is PA282761.

The Life Aquatic with Steve Zissou is a 2004 motion picture created by Wes Anderson and Noah Baumbach for the production company Touchstone Pictures, an a.d.o. [alternative designation of] Disney Enterprises, Inc. and it is directed by Wes Anderson. It is owned by Walt Disney Studios. Its Copyright Number is PA1250646.

The Prisoner of Second Avenue is a 1975 motion picture created by Neil Simon for the production company Warner Bros Inc. and it is directed by Melvin Frank. It is owned by Warner Bros Inc. Its Copyright Number is LP44320.

Any and all music lyrics quoted are the copyrighted work of the artist(s) named and identified. They are also produced hereon in under the legal principle of fair dealing under Intellectual Property legislation (UK) and fair use under Section 107 of the Copyright Act (US).

About The Author

Leonard McClane is the ‘pen name’ for a professional investigator in the North-East of England and who has worked in the field for over 25 years in various sectors. He built up and sold one of the most acclaimed investigation and surveillance services in the region then parlayed his professional experience, his obsessive love of movies and "bad" music, and his interest in writing into creating the 'Jake Lehman' trilogy.

The 'Jake Lehman' series is well-received irreverent takes on private eye tropes and mystery novels all shot through with a darkly comedic slant, whilst mining real cases McClane himself has worked on AND skewering real current issues affecting society today. The end result for each book in the 'Jake Lehman' series - Lehman's Terms, Lehman's Run and Lehman's Infamy - is stories told in a way he hopes no one has experienced.

Leonard is happily married with two children and lives in Newcastle upon Tyne. He is a successful and respected speaker on the subject of professional investigation and has featured in international teaching textbooks regarding raising skills in the investigatory field.

He is also too frequently mistaken for his fictional creation, 'Jake Lehman'. You can follow Leonard McClane on Twitter ('X') at @leonard_mcclane. For any enquiries about him or The Yippee Kai-Yay Principle you can contact the publishing arm Underdog Day at underdogday@outlook.com.

"... Can't win 'em all."

"You'd like to win one though, wouldn't you?"

"One... would be nice!"

Printed in Great Britain
by Amazon

53266030R00175